Then Came Life

Living with Courage, Spirit, and Gratitude after Breast Cancer

GERALYN LUCAS

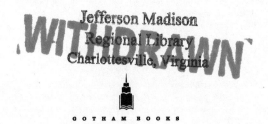

GOTHAM BOOKS

30691 3854

L

GOTHAM BOOKS
Published by the Penguin Group
Penguin Group (USA) LLC
375 Hudson Street
New York, New York 10014, USA

USA | Canada | UK | Ireland | Australia
New Zealand | India | South Africa | China
penguin.com
A Penguin Random House Company

LIBRARY OF CONGRESS CATALOGING-IN-PUBLICATION DATA
Lucas, Geralyn.
Then came life : living with courage, spirit, and gratitude after breast cancer /
Geralyn Lucas.
pages cm
ISBN 978-1-592-40895-5
1. Lucas, Geralyn—Health.   2. Breast—Cancer—Patients—
United States—Biography.   I. Title.
RC280.B8L828 2014
616.99'4490092—dc23
[B]
2014014688

Printed in the United States of America
1   3   5   7   9   10   8   6   4   2

Set in Adobe Garamond Pro
Designed by Spring Hoteling

For Skye Meredith Lucas: Thank you for making me believe in life again and for reminding me to never forget that the sky is the limit.

For Tyler: Thank you for your love and support, and for Skye and Hayden.

For Nilas, Darci, Ripley, Stella, Scarlett, Ruby, Dahlia, Sasha: So glad I got to meet you.

For Harvey and Barbara for starting it all . . .

And to my doctors and nurses for helping me reach this day: Dr. Steven T. Brower, Dr. Anne Moore, Dr. Alisan Estabrook, Dr. Rhoda Sperling, Dr. Susan R. Droffman, Dr. Jill Fishbane-Mayer, Dr. Lyris A. Schonholz, Dr. Len Horovitz, Dr. Sandra Haber, Dr. H. David Goodman, Dr. Kevin Fox, and the Oncology Nursing Society for all the healers you have trained.

CONTENTS

CONTENTS

Life can only be understood backwards; but it must be lived forwards.

Søren Kierkegaard

Sometimes your only available transportation is a leap of faith.

Margaret Shepard

Then Came Life

CHAPTER 1
Right Now: Stop and Smell the Roses

I talk too much. Mostly to myself.

Sometimes the conversations are productive pep talks, but usually they are negative and don't reflect how optimistic I want to be and all the money I spend on therapy and that I am a cancer survivor and I'm still alive.

I was only twenty-seven years old when I was diagnosed with a very aggressive breast cancer. Because of my age and the type of cancer, the prognosis wasn't great: They expected me to have a recurrence within two years, and any future recurrence would more than likely be, as they said, "treatable," not "curable." Every six months I'd have blood tests to check my tumor levels; I was constantly put into different scanning machines so the doctors could look at all my organs to make sure the cancer hadn't traveled somewhere else. A single rogue cell could start trouble again.

I'm forty-five now, but I remember when all I wanted was to hit thirty. At the time that seemed like a more dignified age to die than twenty-eight or twenty-nine. I had read the statistics for the percentages of women who would be alive two years, five years after my kind of diagnosis. Even though I survived the first round with cancer—six months of chemotherapy and a mastectomy—I never knew if or when there might be another round. Would I die or live? Which column would I land in?

When I turned forty, my forty-year-old friends started complaining that we were getting old. I always thought: *Please don't complain to me about getting old; I know the other option too well.* Each year passed with the punctuation of tests, mammograms, and scary reminders of the possibilities. I still think about those statistics and hold my breath every time I wait for my medical test results. All that worrying—and then came life.

For instance: Tonight I'm on my way to Saratoga Springs for my seven-year-old son's chess tournament. We are all squeezed into the car, three moms and three sons. We have already been pulled over by the cops for making a left turn from the right lane. It wasn't really our fault; the GPS isn't working. I am sandwiched in the backseat between two boys playing video games. The games are loud, there's not enough heat, and I wish I weren't in this car. The conversation has begun, and I'm so relieved that the other moms and kids can't hear what I'm saying to myself.

You're dreading the weekend. Chess moms are so uptight. After he lost a round, last year, Hayden complained that you don't push him hard enough to practice, and that he wants you to be a Tiger Mom. You don't even remember how to play checkers or backgammon.

I interrupt the conversation and ask Hayden to turn the music down so I can hear myself better. I pull out my mirror that lights up in the dark and stare at myself.

Your hair is so gray—you haven't had time to dye it. Why do you always revert to pulling it back in a greasy ponytail?

I squint into the mirror to see better in the dark and realize how much my face is falling. My Botox shot is long overdue. My pants are too tight. I unbutton them so I can breathe. I pull my sweater down to cover my muffin top.

Maybe you didn't need those fries with your meal today. Aren't you trying to be healthier?

I have no cute clothes anymore. Earlier today when I was packing, I sneaked into my teenage daughter's room to borrow a T-shirt. She claims my stomach stretches her shirts, so I'm not allowed to wear her cute stuff. She scares me. She's the cool girl I never was. I worry about our relationship lately. She seems like she hates me.

I want to call Tyler from the car, but I figure he'll just screen the call. I can't remember the last time we had a real conversation.

I feel all the gratitude for my hard-earned life draining out of me. All the things I wanted so desperately, clung to life so I could keep, just feel like a drag at this moment. I sigh into the mirror.

. . . . .

Before they wheeled me into the OR, I put on bright red lipstick and I swore to myself that I would come out the other side and become the woman I never thought I could be. I would dare to live up to my lipstick and make every day red-lipstick-worthy. It was all about transformation: As my breast was being removed, I was going to be glamorous and reinvent myself. I had always been a gloss girl, and I thought I couldn't wear red like other women. But I decided to wear bright red lipstick to my mastectomy to show the doctors and nurses in the operating room that I had places to go, things to do. And here I am in the car nineteen years later, a chess mom. Alive.

I pull out a new tube of red lipstick and pucker up.

You need a lip wax.

It's going to be hard to put the lipstick on right at sixty-five miles per hour, but I need to live up to that notice-me hyper-red lipstick again. I need to make that feeling last, to remember the courage from that morning in the operating room and have it inform my entire life. No more taking life for granted.

I pause to reflect, and a different voice chimes in to the conversation in my head:

Remember when you thought you'd never have kids after cancer? This little guy is your bonus. Remember when he was in speech therapy and couldn't pronounce an *R* and you worried about his future? Now he's playing two-hour notated games. And your hair—remember when it all fell out from chemotherapy? When you used to watch Hair Club for Men commercials and cry? Remember when shampoo commercials made you lustful? You prayed to grow old when you were only twenty-seven and diagnosed with cancer. You said all you wanted were wrinkles—and now you hate them? And yeah, so you've gained a few pounds. At least you're healthy. Do you remember when you had to drink Ensure to keep your weight up for the chemotherapy treatments? How can you be afraid of your own daughter? And so grumpy at Tyler? He was there when you woke up from your mastectomy. Why do you fight all the time if you were strong enough to survive cancer together? What else could be so bad?

You are *lucky* to be alive. To be a mom, to have hair, to have wrinkles. How dare you take one day for granted. Remember the friends you met who weren't as lucky, who would give anything to be here, alive.

I take a deep and grateful inhale to slow down and smell the roses in my life. Long breath in through my nose, long exhale from my mouth. A cleansing breath. Breathing connects me to life. It is at this precise moment that my son and his friends begin to have a farting contest.

"Guys, *gross*!" I yell, and they all crack up.

I am trying to smell the roses, but all I can smell are the farts in the car. I lean across my son and hit the button to put the back window down as fast as possible.

"Mom, you have a double chin, like *Family Guy*. I'm sorry, Mom, it's true." Hayden is giving me the news as I'm trying to jut my face out the window to suck in the fresh air.

Sometimes gratitude is so easy for me. Other times it's hard, like when I'm bored, cold, and grossed-out. I have everything I worried I never would, and it came with more heartache and pain and gray hair and wrinkles and cellulite and insomnia and even more joy than I ever imagined.

I'm not going to take one day of life for granted. I promise.

I keep inhaling. I'm visualizing my roses, even though the farts are lingering. The roses are long-stemmed and fragrant, not like the corner-market kind that have no scent. Mine are perfumed, and a reminder of how gorgeous life can be, how you can miss it if you don't pause and reflect, appreciate, and see what is right in front of you as life whizzes by.

My son is laughing hysterically, even as I'm almost crying because his farts are so bad.

Be grateful.

Okay, it's hard to be grateful for farts. But I need to remember to cherish it all, even the farts!

We arrive at the hotel. I smile at my son in the badly fluorescent-lit corridor of check-in. Hayden seems concerned and points at my mouth. I have lipstick on my teeth.

I'm not sure if he's embarrassed by me or looking out for me, but

I wipe my teeth quickly and do a lipstick check with him: thumbs-up.
I decide it's his way of showing me he loves me.

Chess: game on.

Life: game on.

Here is my story of mining the gratitude.

Chapter 2
Skye's the Limit

*M*y name is Geralyn Lucas, and I have a shopping problem. I have always had a shopping problem.

Admitting it is the first step to recovery.

It got worse after my cancer diagnosis. Not only was I looking to replace my lost nipple with every purchase, but shopping took on a deeper meaning. Shopping was a way of running toward life, a declaration that I was sticking around: I needed to *wear* all the purchases. Buying stuff guaranteed more time: I was *shopping*, not dying.

The things I bought seemed to promise a new identity, novel experiences, and possible life-changing opportunities. A new me was always just a purchase away. Hiding my shopping bags from my husband, Tyler, was a full-time job. Tyler would ask, "Is that a new dress?"

"No, I've had this forever. You don't remember?"

Even chemo couldn't keep me from shopping. After my injections, feeling woozy, nauseated, exhausted, veins blackened, I always found just enough energy to make it to T. J. Maxx. Plus, losing my hair opened up a whole new shopping category: I was suddenly in the market for berets, baseball hats, fedoras, and scarves. No one could judge me for buying new head coverings; they were an essential part of my self-esteem. Did I really need four fedoras? Or eleven baseball caps, in every color, smooth velvet and plush velvet, wool and satin? Yeah, I did; the berets would bring a sophistication that had always eluded me, the baseball caps a downtown edge I had craved.

After spending time with the skull and crossbones on my chemo bag, wheeled over to me on the IV pole, shopping felt so *alive*. I had places to go, people to meet, *things to wear*.

"I shop, therefore I exist."

One day, after an especially awful chemo when they couldn't find a "good" vein and had to reinsert the needle three times, I fled to the warm and reassuring shopping aisles of T. J. It was only when I was at the checkout counter, surveying my loot, planning all the different outfits that would coordinate with my new hats, that I had an existential moment of sorts. Just as I was about to swipe my credit card, a voice inside my head boomed so loudly that I was sure the cashier could hear it too.

You can't take it with you.

People could be buried in their favorite outfits, but there was no way that I could wear all these hats at once to my funeral. I didn't know how to explain all this to the cashier, so I bought everything anyway, but as I unpacked at home I had that sickening and paralyzing thought again: I couldn't take it with me.

Where exactly would all my prized possessions go?

Before I could spend too much time worrying about that, I had more stuff. After chemo my hair grew into a chemo-chic short buzz-cut look, and none of my old clothing matched my hair. My wardrobe was too conservative. I needed edgier suits to match my hair. And then there was my chest. Two A-cups had become a removed-then-reconstructed B-plus-cup, and the other one enhanced to match, thanks to my plastic surgeon. So of course I needed new bras. It was nice to have a medical excuse to shop: It felt like having a prescription that said "Go shopping" instead of a prescription for a dose of medication. I did need an entire new wardrobe after my cancer treatments, and I was ready. My look was evolving. Tyler bought me a black satin suit with zippers, to match my new punk hair. I was trying to forge a new identity for my new life. I loved feeling so new and different, like maybe the cancer couldn't find *me* again.

But I worried a lot about the cancer coming back. I developed a phobia about waiting. I couldn't wait in lines at the bank. Tyler tried to take me to an art exhibit to cheer me up on a really bad day, and I had to leave because of the crowd. It got so bad that I had to go on medication. I went to a doctor who specialized in EMDR, a kind of therapy used for people who have suffered severe trauma and PTSD, and I began to understand that I had a fear of waiting because I thought I didn't have enough time left until my cancer might return. Waiting for *anything* reminded me of being in doctors' waiting rooms, waiting for bad news. Waiting for test results, watching the second hand on the big clock as I waited to get my bone scan. Minutes in machines felt like hours; days waiting for blood-test results to see if my tumor levels were up and my cancer was back were torture. My doctor prescribed Zoloft to take the OCD edge off my cancer-returning ruminations. It helped with my worrying, but nothing soothed me like being let loose at a T. J. Maxx. Spending time in the home-goods section was better than a double dose of Zoloft. Looking at linens, shopping for pots and pans, buying another ceramic rooster, just brought a sense of calm that maybe I had a future.

I became a big returner of gifts because that gave me a chance to shop again, without guilt, and it seemed there was always something better out there just calling my name loudly. Returning was a guilt-free shop—found money that I could spend on something new.

After all the anguish, I made it to thirty, and got fantastic birthday presents. The "Now that you have cancer, let me show you how much I love you" presents. I was drooling over one particular present-return because the gift came from a store that was way out of my league, a store that had a doorbell, plush carpeting, and in which—when I walked in—it was clear from what I was wearing that I did not belong. The only reason I was holding a shopping bag from that store was to return something. I did have awkward return-guilt, and was extremely self-conscious to go to such a fancy store. I knew the drill: Fancy stores have the worst return rules and are real sticklers. I reassured myself that it was ridiculous to be intimidated by a store, and especially not a fashion-model-look-alike sales associate named Candy, who inspected me as I handed over the bag.

"Return?" She was glaring at me like I was ungrateful, and her stare seemed to say, "Do you know how much time we spent looking for the perfect present for you, scouring the store? Your friend thought you would love the shirt. If she could see you now, she might cry."

To make matters worse, the birthday card was still in the box. It had a heart drawn on the envelope, with my name above it.

"You forgot something," Candy said with a smirk.

I kept checking to make sure my friend wasn't outside the store looking through the glass and watching me return the present, or standing behind me at the register because she had forgotten something in the store and just happened to be there at the precise moment I decided to come in and return the present. I imagined the expression on her face when she realized I hadn't come to find a pair of pants that matched the shirt she had painstakingly picked out. Is there return-karma? I felt it burning shame into my red face. I wanted to blurt, "I know it's not the present, it's the thought that counts, but I only wanted to shop more." I was a lowlife. I had taken her beautiful sentiment, her act of caring, and made it a cold, hard business calculation.

Any return-guilt evaporated when the salesgirl handed me the receipt. I knew I had to act calm when I saw the credit. I nearly screamed, "She paid that for *that*?" but fortunately my return experience came in handy and I just glanced at the receipt calmly. "Why don't you look around?" Candy suggested. "We just got some great pieces in."

Before I could start browsing, something flashy and sparkling winked at me from a glass case across the store. I tried to head toward the sweaters, but that thing kept flirting: Sparkling red and pink gemstones were luring me toward the glass case. I couldn't turn away. Candy noticed the seduction going down and came over to make a formal introduction. She took out a set of keys to remove a jeweled cowboy belt from its case. When she held it in her hands, it seemed to sparkle even more outside its case in the direct store light.

"It's like a piece of jewelry, isn't it? Handmade, so much craftsmanship." Candy looked like she wanted the belt too. "Do you want to hold it?"

Hold it? I was almost scared to touch it.

"Look: It has sterling-silver trim, traditional cowboy style, with all these semiprecious gemstones." The stones made a dazzling pattern and the sparkle-wattage had us under its spell. It was a tiara version of a cowboy belt, with ruby red and the prettiest pink and vibrant violet crystals encrusting the belt, and the buckle was the most tasteful design ever. The silver seemed to make the crystals shine even more.

"Try it on," Candy encouraged me.

I was experiencing the ultimate shopping moment. This belt had the potential to transform me into a person I never thought I could be. This belt was red lipstick on steroids. This belt was self-actualization. This belt would make me live forever. I would jump out of my convertible wearing the belt. I don't have a car and I don't drive, but the belt would make me just that daring. The belt would make me a world traveler; it would encourage me to visit its relatives in Austria, where I could buy more crystal-laden things. I could buy Austrian-crystal chandelier earrings and real chandeliers, and I could hop over to Italy because it's right on the border. The belt would encourage me to stay thin because it accented my waist. Actually, it wouldn't matter how much I weighed, because the beauty of the belt would distract people. By association, I would be prettier.

My hands were a bit sweaty as I looped the belt through my jeans. Candy had to help me because I was shaking so much. I had never owned anything like this, and when I looked at myself in the mirror, I sort of hallucinated the new life that awaited me.

The belt was reminding me of everything I wanted. I imagined brunches where I would never wait for a table because the belt had seduced the hostess. The belt would be a magnet, drawing to me all the perfect things that had never been attracted to me before. The belt was the perfect combination of high and low fashion. It was as glamorous as a high heel, but as practical as a flat. And where exactly was I going to wear this crystal cowboy belt? Well, everywhere. I could dress it up or dress it down. I knew this belt would bring me invitations to places where it would look perfect. It seemed like the kind of belt Pink might own. She would wear it to her recording studio. It would be so dazzling that it might inspire a new song. Women who would wear this belt were rock stars. This was a belt that conveyed a lifestyle, and new horizons would be discovered wearing this belt.

To make the belt even better, it had to be special-ordered from Austria, where all the crystals would be hand-applied. The one I tried on was a store model.

Candy explained, "It should take about three weeks for your belt to arrive." Each dazzling crystal, shining brighter than I could dream, would be placed precisely into *my* belt. The wait was hard because I wanted the life that would come with it. Before the belt arrived, I had a strange dream that my nipple, the one I lost in my mastectomy, materialized from Austria. How did it ever find its way back to me? But when I woke up, I started craving the real package I was waiting for.

Finally the belt arrived. Candy called and sounded so excited on the phone.

"It's here, and I think it's even shinier than the floor model!"

Call-waiting was beeping through. My doctor's office. I didn't want to leave the belt's status hanging there for even a moment.

"Candy, I'm so sorry, it's my doctor's office." I clicked over. I always had to take calls from my doctor.

Line one seemed to be the new life, just imported from Austria. Line two: It could be cancer.

I was three weeks pregnant.

Doctors had told me I would go into early menopause because of chemotherapy. I couldn't bank eggs before chemo because the doctors were worried that the hormones would jump-start any rogue cancer cells. I begged, but they wouldn't relent. They told me I needed to wait at least two years after treatment before trying to get pregnant to make sure that my cancer wasn't coming back.

There was no consensus on whether it was safe to get pregnant after breast cancer. But one thing doctors did agree on: If I got pregnant, I would be a high-risk patient; the baby and I would have to be monitored closely.

At the time I was a story editor at the newsmagazine show *20/20*, and I went straight into research mode. I found the preeminent Dr. P, studying the question "How safe is it for a young woman to get pregnant after breast cancer?" Unfortunately, her study—announced in the journal *Cancer*—found that pregnancy after breast cancer was *not* as safe as previously assumed.

I contacted Dr. P anyway. She said, "If I were you, I'd adopt."

I understood that getting pregnant was filled with risk. If I got cancer while I was pregnant, there was a program in Texas in which women could have chemotherapy after the third month, because after that the chemicals wouldn't cross the placenta and injure the baby. But then I was haunted by the question: What if I had a baby and then I went and died on her? What if I died before I could teach her anything?

A piece I was working on at *20/20* finally convinced me that having a baby was still worth a shot. The story was about Erin, a mom whose daughter Peyton was only four years old when she started videotaping a farewell to her child because she was dying of breast cancer. At first Erin was scared to tape her good-bye, but once she started, she couldn't stop. She talked about everything from what to say to boys to what to do when Dad remarried, and how much she loved Peyton. Erin showed me that I could still be a mom no matter what, and that love was so much stronger than cancer. And I can't describe how badly I wanted a baby. Put every purse, every shoe, every pair of jeans, every necklace I had drooled over in a huge pile and it wouldn't compare to how much I wanted to be a mom. It was a longing unlike any I had ever experienced. The more they told me it was impossible, the more I wanted to be a mom. I had always wanted to be a mom, ever since I was little and played with dolls. Now I wanted it even more because I'd had cancer.

One rogue cancer cell started all my trouble, and one rogue sperm was responsible for my impending joy: Thank you, Tyler! Having a baby after cancer felt like a sprint toward life. There was no turning back if you were pushing a baby carriage.

When I clicked back over to Candy, I was still crying tears of joy about my baby news. Maybe one tear of lament: the belt. I tried to imagine if I could wear the belt while I was pregnant. How long did pregnant women retain any waistline? Could I have the belt expanded? But I'd never seen a pregnant woman actually wearing a belt.

"Candy, this is so awkward. The belt. Can I return it? I'm pregnant!"

"No problem; in fact, I just had a woman who wanted one too. Come into the store; we just got some great new things that might be more practical." The word "practical" hung in the air, and every dream about the belt and me evaporated and was replaced with visions of diapers, burp cloths, bottles, baby wipes, and the smell of poopy and spit-up. Those visions almost choked me when I returned to the store. I saw the belt one more time in its case, working its wiles on me again.

Candy led me away from the case toward a black sweater made with spandex. She explained it would stretch comfortably around my expanding belly and then shrink back after my pregnancy. The good news: I had a whole new category of shopping to do—maternity wear.

·   ·   ·   ·

*A*nd once I realized I was having a girl, it was off to the baby stores because she *needed* that adorable leopard-print onesie. Shopping for baby clothing is an unfair challenge to someone with a shopping issue. Baby clothes are all too cute and irresistible, and it's always practical to keep buying stuff, because babies grow so fast! My daughter had black-fur-lined white go-go boots (bought on deep discount), before she could even walk, actually before she was born.

I named my baby for the mantra that had sustained me through every surgery, every IV they put into me. My hypnotherapist had suggested the mantra. Here's what she said: "You are like the sky. Nothing can stick to you, not even a needle. The sky is vast and open and never changes, even though there are changes. A plane can roar through the sky, a storm, a sunrise, and a sunset. You can throw paint at the sky, and it will always be the sky." I was safe because I was the sky, so I named my daughter Skye.

My estimated due date: July 26, the exact date I'd had my biopsy four years before. How could the same date mean such different things? A diagnosis of malignant cells and a birth. Was that a bad omen or a good omen? The baby would just miss having Cancer as her astrological sign—I had forgotten that cancer could also be *a* Cancer, a baby born when the sun was in that sign of the zodiac. Her life was a new symbol of life for me: Those endless white hospital floors had led me to the operating room for surgery to remove cancer, and now they'd take me to the OR for a C-section to give me a baby.

I wore lipstick to my C-section.

It was surreal to wear lipstick in the very same hospital, to a very similar operating room, for such a different reason. When I had put on lipstick four years earlier, I never imagined wearing lipstick to meet my baby daughter.

Tyler was there in the OR, as he was for my mastectomy. When we heard our daughter's first cry of life, it seemed to dry the tears we'd both cried before. He assured me that he would be both daddy and mommy if my cancer came back. He knew that having a baby with me was a risk, but he wanted to take it. "I want your baby so I'll always have a piece of you if anything goes wrong."

Remarkably, her eyes were sky blue, sparkling brighter than Austrian crystals, rimmed with thick black natural-mascara lashes. She, like my mantra, would heal me. Her middle name was Meredith, to add more gravitas and to honor my former boss, who survived breast cancer but was never able to have a child. Giving my baby the name Skye Meredith was my tribute to the journey I took to have her. She could always be S. Meredith if she wanted to be a lawyer or do something else serious.

In the hospital she was brought to me in a little glass jewel box; the nurse wheeled her in, like wheeling in room service. The box was like a present from Tiffany's—all that was missing was a satin bow.

Her skin was pink and soft and suddenly she was the best present ever. This was better than my engagement ring. Better than the black patent-leather shoes I looked at in the window longingly for three weeks waiting for them to go on sale. Better than the Austrian crystal cowboy belt. Anything I had ever wanted before seemed to go to the bottom of my wish list, and she was on the top. I loved Skye in a way I had never loved anyone or anything before. Just saying I loved her didn't seem enough.

The glass box was so clear, I could see through it perfectly, and so clear there were no reflections to distract from the main attraction. This glass held no secrets and it was shiny like her new life. It was the perfect glass to hold her, like a simple clear glass vase to showcase only the beauty of the flower it's holding. I just wanted to stare at her in there. When she was returned to the nursery, there was a glass wall between us, a glass wall marked with the fingerprints and breath of parents pushing up against it to look at these babies all wrapped in blankets.

Sometimes I'd look in on her in the middle of the night, staring at her until I needed to shuffle back to my room, barely able to stand from the C-section, to take painkillers. But the painkillers didn't kill the pain I felt from being away from her while she was sleeping in the nursery. I needed to be with her, next to her, all the time. On my second night in the hospital, I pulled myself slowly to the nursery, holding on to the wall to keep my balance. When I got there I expected to see Skye sleeping peacefully in her blanket. She was screaming.

"I will rescue you. I will know when you're crying," I said to myself in a low but firm voice so the other people standing at the glass wouldn't think I was talking to myself like a crazy woman. "I will know whenever you cry; I will be your knight in my hospital gown, here to rescue you, my princess in your poopy diaper." It was so strange and complicated—this love I felt for her despite morning sickness and vomiting, three days of labor, the cut from the C-section that seemed to hurt especially when I held her, the breast-feeding on one boob. All of that risk to have her was rewarded by staring into her blue eyes, feeling invincible, like my mantra: "I am the sky."

My twenty-nine-year-old cousin Hallie came to visit me in the hospital when Skye was born. She had no kids of her own, but she held Skye expertly, like she was holding a box marked FRAGILE. Then she sang her a Madonna song called "Little Star." Madonna had written the song about her own daughter's birth and how much it meant to her after losing her mom when she was just five, to breast cancer. Hallie was so thoughtful that way. She knew the song was about healing after a loss, and how a baby could do that. She was also showing me that Madonna had grown up after the loss of her mom and become Madonna: Skye would be okay if she lost me.

And she would have Tyler. He promised to be there for her if I got sick. After I got out of the hospital and went back to work, I was exhausted from working all the time and staying up at night with Skye. Tyler was amazing. He was such a competent dad. I always put the diapers on a bit lopsided; he did them with surgical precision. He loved taking naps with Skye asleep on his chest and country music playing in the background. Tyler even learned the Teletubby dance for Skye.

He was much better than I was at being a parent with rules. The only thing we disagreed about was the pacifier: He wanted it gone and I didn't. I think I wanted to be especially nice to Skye so that if I died she could remember that I had let her do anything. I kept a few pacifiers hidden just in case she needed one. When she was teething, she wanted to chomp on everything, and it felt as if she were taking a big bite out of life. People tried to explain to me how much I would love my child. They told me that it would overwhelm me and be an experience I'd never had before. It was as if all the love I'd ever felt for any shopping conquest was shamed. Her arrival trumped the nipple I'd lost.

I still can't describe the love I have for that little girl. I still lust for things and I still have a problem with shopping. Whoever said the best things in life couldn't be bought is just a little bit wrong; there are still a lot of things I just *need*. Yes, I have a problem. But in addition to having an entirely new shopping category, I have a new life category too.

I dream occasionally about the crystal belt and the life we would have had together, but I have a new belt now. Where the belt would have sat on my waist there's a little ridge now from the C-section I had. It's my second large scar, this C-section scar, on the opposite side of my mastectomy scar. The mastectomy scar meant something was taken away; the C-section scar meant I had been given something. Death and life were just inches away on the road map of my body.

Every time I look down at my stomach, exactly where the cowboy belt would have gleamed with pure Austrian crystals, I think how lucky I am to be wearing this C-section belt instead. Having a baby after breast cancer meant that I had tricked the cancer by creating a new life. Somehow my body grew a new life instead of a new tumor. It was a huge leap of faith, starting a new life when mine felt so shaky. I felt like I had crossed a finish line by having Skye after cancer, but I didn't realize that I was actually starting an entirely new marathon: motherhood.

CHAPTER 3
Killer Butt

*P*eople say that writing a book is like having a baby. I was trying to do both at once: While I was nursing Skye with one boob, changing her diapers, and getting blood tests and other scans to make sure my cancer hadn't returned, I was also setting my alarm clock for four A.M. to work on my book. I was obsessed with nurturing my babies: Skye and my book.

At my book party, five-year-old Skye was like a mini-me, wearing the exact same outfit that I was—her little jeans had a stretchy back, her Betsey Johnson T-shirt was a scaled-down version of mine that I'd had made at the tailor, and we both had bright pink feather boas.

I wanted to give hope to other women, but maybe more importantly I wanted to inform them. Especially young women, because I was still in shock over what had happened to me at only twenty-seven with no known family history. I had thought that for me to get breast cancer, my mom had to have had it. I had thought I had to be at least forty. Probably fifty, sixty, or seventy. I was a journalist, working at ABC News, pitching medical stories, and I still didn't know the basic facts about breast cancer: Most women who get breast cancer don't have a family history, and women in their twenties and thirties can get it too—and are often misdiagnosed because they're told they are "too young."

Lipstick was a big part of my story. The book was even titled *Why I Wore Lipstick to My Mastectomy*. It was published in 2004. When I held the first book in my hand, I thought that I had written the book I'd needed to read when I was diagnosed: I wanted someone to tell me the truth about having a mastectomy, about chemo, about reconstruction, or that losing a breast could mean losing a nipple too. Right after my reconstruction surgery, my doctors asked me to do a show-and-tell with women all over New York City, so they could see what my reconstructed breast looked like in a bra; I let the women touch my breast to see what it felt like too. Writing my book was a big overshare—a way to help even more women get through it.

It was the morning of my first official book signing, different from my book party, which was just for friends and family. I was obsessing about what to wear over my Spanx. What do authors wear to book signings? I wanted to look like my author photo, but it was severely airbrushed. I looked nothing like the woman in the photo: wind-blown raven hair, eyes that sparkled without a hint of exhaustion, and perfectly flawless skin. I had worked so hard to make my book authentic, and my cover photo was blowing it. The usual me was in a greasy ponytail, with a touch of adult acne, and wearing eye concealer that clashed with my actual skin tone.

It wasn't that easy, wearing that Spanx. First, I had to get it on. There was panting and bucking and first I got into one leg, and then I almost toppled over but pulled up the other leg. The horizon was in front of me and all I had to do was get the Spanx over my butt. I lay down on the bed, breathed in and pulled, then jumped off the bed squatting and wobbling like a penguin. I then did a modified rain dance to hike it fully over my hips. It got stuck on my kidney, or my liver. Can Spanx do organ damage? When I finally got it over my last little C-section hump I wondered: Whom exactly was I putting this Spanx on for? Why did I need to look smoother, smaller, or better for someone else? I mean, I knew I was wearing the Spanx. My husband, Tyler, knew I was wearing Spanx, so wasn't it really a bit disingenuous? Would someone like my book better because of the Spanx?

I hurt a finger on my right hand, my *signing* hand, getting into that Spanx. I had imagined how gracefully an author might autograph her book at her first signing, and exactly the curly *G* I wanted to make in my name, and now my finger was pounding and felt sprained. How could I sign all those books? Was it a sign about losing my self-respect in the process?

The Spanx had one last little roar left: It rolled down when I exhaled, and my stomach popped over it. Me versus Spanx. Spanx, first round.

I had been told that I would be speaking to seven hundred women at Women's Health and Fitness Expo at the Javits Center. Seven hundred people! I didn't *know* that many people. At Javits, on my way down the escalator to my room, I saw different ads for different seminars, all relating to the "wellness" theme. Women attending the programs could choose either my seminar or another seminar being held at the same time. I was scheduled for 4:00 P.M. It was 3:50. The media escort had told me they were expecting full capacity. Possible overflow! I tried to muster my courage. I reminded myself that I had won the Optimist Award in eleventh grade. I had to try to smile like the book jacket and pretend I really felt like an author.

And then I saw the competition. Well, actually, I saw her sign first: KILLER BUTT! Thank goodness I had worn a Spanx. I knew that women at this convention would be taking their bodies seriously, but I'd never dreamed there'd be a class called "KILLER BUTT!" I knew about core, crunches, squats, but how cool that there was a specific class about how to get a KILLER BUTT!, all caps with an exclamation point. There was a video called *Buns of Steel*, but something about the "KILLER BUTT!" was so in-your-face, so intimidating, and so serious. As if after the class the instructor's butt might actually kill someone.

I wasn't the only woman who was intrigued. As the escalator continued down, I kept twisting my neck to watch the video loop that was playing next to the KILLER BUTT! sign. A line of women watched the video outside the room, and there was quite a bit of commotion inside the room too.

I tripped over the bottom landing of the escalator. I should have been headed to my convention room, but I couldn't help walking toward the "KILLER BUTT!" room. The instructor was wearing Lycra, and her goods matched her product. It was round, smooth, firm, and did this strange thing where it seemed to lift up, as if her behind were wearing a push-up bra.

For only $19.99 it could be yours.

Everyone knows breasts and butts rule, but living with one boob, you know it more. Why are there breastaurants named Hooters? I know the chicken wings are good, but . . . And why is there a *Sports Illustrated* swimsuit edition? Why is there a Victoria's Secret "fashion" show? Why did Janet Jackson's nipple-flash launch an FCC investigation? I don't have a nipple anymore. I felt disenfranchised somehow, and "KILLER BUTT!" was hitting the head of my nail of insecurity.

I had a message of hope and courage, but women had their choice of presentations, and I was worried that "KILLER BUTT!" would win. To tell the truth, it *killed me* to miss "KILLER BUTT!"

I checked my watch: 3:56. I was on at four o'clock; I had to get to my room to greet *my* peeps.

As I approached my room, there was no one outside waiting to greet me. No line. No matter. My crowd must be inside, wanting to get the good seats. My crowd was clearly more erudite, more civilized, more cultivated and calm and not fawning over a butt video. My crowd wanted to hear about a triumph of life, about the act of finding courage, about being scared of dying but somehow going forward. I took a very deep sort of yoga breath because we were at the Women's Health and Fitness Expo, and walked into my room. My debut moment of authorness.

Rows and rows and rows of white chairs, without a butt in sight.

I instantly remembered every birthday party I was never invited to, every girl who excluded me, every boy who didn't return a crush. It had to be a mistake. I must have the wrong time and wrong room. I ran out and checked the program again; I looked at the number outside my room to see if it matched. It matched; there was no mistake. This was my room, and I was alone in it. This is what emptiness looks like, rows and rows of chairs with no one in them.

Emptiness feels like no one cares.

Emptiness sounds like silence, and makes any other insignificant noise loud. I could hear the buzzing of the air conditioner system.

I had two compelling thoughts. One: Run up the escalator and pretend I had never come to the book signing, that I'd never tried to be an author. Two: Attend and try to blend in at "KILLER BUTT!" But what if someone in "KILLER BUTT!" saw me and knew I was the author supposed to be giving a lecture about my new book during the same time period? Impossible, I looked nothing like my book jacket.

I blinked and stared hard at the room and the rows of white. The overhead lighting was bright and fluorescent. The room was freezing; I guess they thought all the bodies would have brought the temperature up. At the front of the room was the stage and a huge box of books. And a mic. And a podium. I saw the Sharpie I was supposed to use to sign the books for the people who never came. Should I go up onstage and give my speech anyway? To an empty room? No, I should go back home, be with my daughter. She'd cried when I'd left for this book event, when I told her she had to spend a couple of hours without me.

I was preparing to leave when I saw her—the only woman in the audience. All the way in the back of the room, in the last seat.

My first instinct was to run away. Maybe she would never guess that I was the author. But I took a deep breath, and I did a walk of shame to my lone audience member. Is one even an audience? How should I handle this? I wasn't quite sure of book-signing etiquette. She wasn't even wearing lipstick. She looked as terrified as I felt, but *she* was the one sniffling and crying.

"My name is Geralyn Lucas. Believe it or not, I'm the author. I really don't look anything like my book jacket."

"My name is Janina," she said. "My daughter told me you were going to be here. She sent me this flyer." She held up a piece of paper, with fake me smiling. "I'm having my mastectomy on Thursday, but don't think I can do it. My daughter said we should come. We took the bus four hours to meet you. From Reading, Pennsylvania."

I didn't answer. I couldn't speak.

"That's where I live."

I started to cry, which I was sure wasn't author-like behavior, but I couldn't help myself, because she believed I could help her.

And then I realized something: I had an audience.

I hugged her and told her what I had planned to say on the podium:

"I put on lipstick for my mastectomy. Before that, I'd been a gloss girl. But I wanted to embolden myself, to have something that shouted out to everyone in the operating theater who I was. How brave I was, though I didn't feel brave. When I woke up in the recovery room, my chest was so heavy, my mouth was dry, and I barely knew where I was. And the first thing the nurse said to me was, 'Girl, what brand is that? I can't believe it lasted through a six-hour surgery.' She called the nurses in the ICU to tell them about it. The doctor took my breast; my lipstick lasted. That lipstick was my voice, my rage, my love, my strength. It was me. What I'm trying to say is, they took a body part, but I kept everything that mattered. You will too."

Now I was close enough to be whispering in her ear. Side by side we kept talking, and we talked for two hours, until the Javits employees arrived to close down the room.

I hurried to the front and officially signed my first book. I couldn't curl the *G* as much as I wanted to because my finger still hurt from the Spanx injury.

On Thursday, Janina's daughter sent me photos of her mom on the gurney, clutching my book. What I couldn't see was that she'd drawn a bright red lipstick heart around the breast she was about to lose. My lipstick had inspired her, but somehow she had inspired me more. God had played a funny trick on me. I had written my book with this premise: "If I reach one woman in her moment of suffering, I will feel it was worth it—all of the pain and suffering I had gone through." And there she was: Janina. She told me later that I was the person who pulled her through, because she knew I had done it. The doctors hadn't, the nurses hadn't, but, Janina said, "If you could have a mastectomy, I could too."

I had thought that the mastectomy would be my defining life moment, my moment of greatest courage. But now I knew there were more hurdles to jump. Hurdles that weren't life or death, or in the OR, but absolutely terrifying, almost paralyzing in other ways—like having one desperately crying woman in the audience in a football-field-size room. They say that the journey of a thousand miles begins with one step, but I never understood that; I was always worried about the other 999.99

miles that came after it. I think that Janina helped me understand that first step. In sharing my private struggle, somehow the pain became bigger, and cracked me open. In all that I lost, I gained even more.

I went into the Javits Center room to sign my first book, and I expected to speak. Instead I had to listen. I entered the room defeated, but I left confident.

Then a funny thing happened.

Women across the country started wearing lipstick to their mastectomies, and they Facebooked their pictures to show me. One woman I met at another book signing told me that she'd worn a *tiara* to her mastectomy! How *regal*. And she was *bald* from her chemo. How did she keep it on? I have no idea. It was like the miracle of red lipstick lasting through the six-hour surgery.

Another woman wore stripper tassels to her mastectomy. Yes, she went in swinging. What could the doctor possibly have thought removing those tassels? My favorite: the woman who wore bright red, sexy panties! She fought with the nurse and demanded she be allowed to wear the red panties into the operating room. The nurse refused to bend the rules, and the lingerie-wearing mastectomy patient demanded to see the supervisor. She won. She told me that breaking the "no underwear" rule felt so rebellious, and gave her a sense of power in a powerless situation.

You *go*, girl.

Red lipstick became a symbol that these women connected with. A total state of mind. I knew what that lipstick had meant to me as I was being wheeled into the operating room; still, the impact of it on everyone else shocked me. And then I heard about the "Lipstick Theory." One of the world's pioneering cancer surgeons, the late William Cahan, MD, chief of surgery at Memorial Sloan-Kettering Cancer Center, coined the term. According to Dr. Cahan, he was able to tell if a patient was improving while being treated for cancer if she started wearing her lipstick. "When a woman who is battling cancer starts to put on lipstick, she is on the road to recovery," he said. "It is when the lipstick is on that she has adopted a 'survivor' frame of mind."

Dr. Cahan served on the medical advisory board of a group called Look Good Feel Better, which helps women going through cancer treatments to learn to look like themselves again with makeup and hair-styling guidance offered by volunteer professionals. A tube of lipstick really does hold transformative powers. I attended Look Good Feel Better (LGFB) workshops and I saw the magic of the theory myself. Patients entered weary, tired, and looking sick, and left transformed. Yes, lipstick—and eyebrow pencils and wigs—were applied, but by the time they left, all the women in that room were changed by hope. They looked at themselves in their mirrors and smiled for the first time in a long time.

But the hope of red lipstick wasn't just limited to cancer patients. I started hearing from women who had never had cancer but who finally believed, after reading my book, that they could wear lipstick. It touched something inside of them, and made them believe they could pull it off. Somehow my metamorphosis reminded them of their own journeys and the different wounds they had overcome.

And then the book was turned into a movie. A tall blonde with long, long legs played me, and her butt defined a whole new category of "KILLER." Red lipstick was crazy powerful. When I arrived on the set of *Why I Wore Lipstick to My Mastectomy* in Toronto, the director's assistant's mom had bold red lips. They were, of course, the first thing I noticed. "I read your book last night," she said, "and I had to go to the drugstore to buy a tube."

"What?" I was genuinely stunned, since she looked like a long-time red-lipstick girl.

"*My* red lipstick means I'm finally able to let people look at me.

I'm ready to get noticed." When she smiled, her teeth looked so white. Another benefit of a red lip. "I just left an abusive relationship. I tried to stand it for so long. I want to put myself out there now." Her red was so intentional. Just like my operating room shade. Red lipstick was about becoming the women we never thought we could be.

The spark set off more sparks. The rights to my book sold in Hungary, then Sweden, then Germany, Japan, and even Italy. I started getting booked for speeches, and the organizer would tell me that 700 women were going to come. Yeah, right, that's a good one. Funny thing is, it was usually 765, and they would run out of tickets. Every time I heard from a woman on my website telling me that my book had helped her, I thought that maybe my mom had put her up to it. But my mom didn't know anyone in Brazil!

A department store hosted a book signing for me, with a makeup artist to show women how to wear a bold red lip. A lot of women turned us down; they didn't think they could wear red and were too scared. One woman protested, "I can only wear corals." She was adamant.

"Who said?" The makeup artist was shaking his head, horrified.

"I just know. Red doesn't work on me. Corals."

The makeup artist gave up, and I wondered why that woman was stuck with that image of herself. And if she would ever see herself differently.

I will never forget the faces of the women I saw wearing lipstick for the first time that day at the department store. When they looked in the mirror, they didn't recognize themselves. It was if they had finally appeared in their lives: bright, bold, *look-at-me* red just daring them to step up to it. Red lipstick was a little revolution inside their heads, a spark that let them see themselves differently.

Could any of this have happened without Janina? I think she started some sort of crazy chain reaction. Actually, *she* believed in me before I really believed in myself. After battling breast cancer, could I win the battle with myself? Janina showed up for me, and that prompted me to keep showing up. That connection is something I will never forget.

I wanted to be open to the universe, to trust it after being so let down by cancer, and I let the universe surprise and delight me. And there was another big shock on the way.

CHAPTER 4
Random Acts

*E*verything about being with Skye made me see my life through a new lens of wonder. Skye let me take off my cancer-colored glasses and put on the rose ones again. Watching her take in life made me feel more alive than I'd ever felt. Her first giggle ricocheted around my heart and its echo stayed with me. On Take Your Daughter to Work Day, six-year-old Skye sat at my desk and pretended to answer the phone the way I did: "Lifetime Television, this is Geralyn Lucas's daughter." She wanted to be me so badly that when we bought matching nightgowns, she wanted to wear the "Mommy" one—and she wore it, dragging on the floor, until it was dirty and had a hole worn in it. Skye would take a nap, falling asleep while holding my hair. I couldn't move but I was happy to lie there, staring at her as she slept, her soft little breathing reminding me that we were both alive. I can still picture her clomping around in my high heels, her tiny feet pushed all the way to the front of the shoes, nearly losing her balance.

Being so in love with Skye made me see that I wanted another

GERALYN LUCAS

child, and Skye was always coming home from playdates asking why she couldn't have a brother or a sister. How could I explain to a six-year-old that I couldn't have another baby because it might be too dangerous—that even having her had been a risk? Now she was here and I couldn't take that risk again. I needed to live for her.

As if to answer my uncertainty about life and how fragile it is, and how I shouldn't mess with my miracle, there was front-page news in *The New York Times* about Dr. P, the doctor I needed to ask about the safety of getting pregnant again:

> A cancer researcher known for her investigations into the aftermath of breast cancer surgery, especially its impact on fertility, was killed in an accident in Manhattan on Monday. She was 57 and lived in Bronxville, N.Y. [She] died in surgery, hours after being struck by an ambulette while crossing the street at Second Avenue and 64th Street. At the time, she was on her way to work at Memorial Sloan-Kettering Cancer Center, where she directed the surgical program at the Evelyn H. Lauder Breast Center.

I threw down the paper. I ran to the bathroom and vomited. *She had devoted her life to helping people like me.* How could a cancer doctor die crossing the street?

Another medical journal noted: "[She] was poised to answer several key questions—most notably, the safety of pregnancy after breast cancer treatment."

My gynecologist had been monitoring my ovaries and told me that I could go into premature ovarian failure from the chemo treatments, and that would mean I was being thrown into early menopause. At my next appointment I told my gynecologist that my periods weren't regular. "If you aren't menstruating every month, it isn't a good sign about your fertility. We can do a test to see how fertile you are, to see what your egg quality is."

The test results were terrible. My follicle stimulation hormone (FSH) was way too high: 20.9. *Four* was normal. Three to nine was the target range, and at above ten, most fertility clinics would not consider you as a candidate. "Your brain is working too hard to get you to ovulate, like stepping on the gas again and again when an engine is dead. I'm sorry. It's probably because of the chemo."

After I heard the news, I saw baby carriages everywhere, and I had to remind myself that I was lucky I'd had even one child after chemotherapy. It was too risky, to be exposed to all those pregnancy hormones *again*. They could restimulate any remaining cancer cells. My estrogen level could increase a thousandfold.

I was still being monitored for any sign of the cancer returning. Every six months my life were PET scans, CT scans, blood tests for tumor levels, and physical exams with my oncologist. I had insisted on wearing my high heels during my next routine PET scan. I had never known if I was allowed to wear heels to my scans, so I just kept them on with my surgical gown when I went into the waiting room.

"Nice shoes." The medical technician was admiring my heels.

"Can I wear them in the machine?" I don't even know why I asked.

"Sure, why not." She seemed as happy about it as I was. Looking at my high heels as I stepped onto the machine that held my fate was a small link to the other world I wanted to continue to live in. These machines were like my crystal balls, and I always tried to read the technicians' faces to see if there was good news or bad. They weren't allowed to tell me anything. All I thought about when I lay in the cold, scary darkness was Skye.

After the test, I went for the follow-up appointment with my oncologist. I must have blacked out when she reviewed the test results and told me where the spot was, because for the life of me I couldn't remember where on my body it was. I called her in a frenzy after I left her office. "Where is it again?"

"On your lung. You need to see a lung specialist immediately."

Days later, the lung specialist explained to me that the spot was actually called a "nodule" and that I needed a surgical procedure where they'd crack my rib cage and remove the lung lobe in order to get to the spot they needed to biopsy. "Unfortunately, we can't reach the spot on your lung by putting a scope down your throat because it's too far away. If I were you, I'd go ahead and schedule your lobe removal quickly. Breast cancer often travels to the lung. If we remove it early, you might not even have to do chemo."

My cancer might be back. This time it might only be "treatable," not "curable," since it would have metastasized to a vital organ. When the doctor was telling me this, all I could focus on was the beautiful aqua-colored Turkish rug in his office. It was mesmerizing, a light turquoise with sand-colored accents. I knew that my results were right in front of him, in an open file, but I was suddenly overwhelmed with a desire to buy a rug.

Actually, I wanted to *be* a rug. Rugs didn't get cancer. Rugs didn't need PET scans. When I was first diagnosed with cancer, buildings would make me cry because I knew they would be there so much longer than I would be. I wanted to be a building, strong as concrete. I wanted to be anything but a medical chart with bad news, another diagnosis. It felt so undignified to be only a diagnosis in front of this man.

"Recovery from this procedure is about six weeks to six months, to get your range of breathing back. Most people don't notice missing a lung lobe. You can still do normal athletic activity," he said.

"Where did you get this rug?"

"My wife picked it out," he said. "It may be hard to talk or even breathe right after surgery, but we can help you with that. Do you understand what I've been saying?"

"Could we call your wife and ask her where she got it?" I wanted to be an inanimate object, completely solid in time and space, so nothing could change. The doctor wanted to schedule my lung lobe removal ASAP. I wanted to head down to ABC Carpet and go rug shopping, and I knew that I had my priorities straight. I wanted to run toward life and keep shopping, not get more bad news.

"You could just watch and wait, though I don't recommend it. But we could send you for another image in, say, six months, and if the nodule looks the same, we could continue to image it and make sure it isn't growing. But if it's cancer, it would spread quickly. I wouldn't take that risk."

That night the doctor's words echoed in my brain as I looked at Skye breathing. She had fallen asleep next to me, holding my hair. Her little chest was moving up and down. I loved her so much that I cried when I clipped her fingernails. I wanted her to feel safe. She'd never seen me sick or in a hospital. I had lost a breast, my hair, and now possibly I'd lose a lung lobe. I spoke with a woman who'd had the same thing happen to her. She'd had her lung lobe removed, and when they did the biopsy on the node, it was breast cancer that had traveled into her lung. She didn't need chemo, and felt she had saved her life. I started thinking about the lipstick I would wear to my lung lobe removal.

But I started worrying they hadn't found it in time. Lately I'd felt a little short of breath. I was due for blood work anyway to measure my tumor levels again. And something else really weird was going on. I couldn't stop eating, more than my normal can't-stop-eating. I was craving a hot open-faced turkey sandwich dripping with gravy, oozing stuffing, and topped with a puddle of cranberry sauce—and it was July. After I ate the sandwich and wanted another one, I realized that the last time I'd felt this way was after chemo. And one other time: when I was pregnant. But now when I pee on three pregnancy sticks, all three tests were negative.

My doctor called me: She had taken blood to test my tumor levels, but there was more news.

"You *are* pregnant. . . ."

But my tumor markers were way up, which meant the cancer was back. Was it the node on my lung? I hadn't scheduled the lobe removal yet; I was waiting. Any joy that I felt about the baby news was trumped by cancer. There was hysteria from my doctors over whether it was medically sound to keep the baby. What if I had cancer and my pregnancy fueled the new cancer? As a doctor himself, Tyler was scared at first, and he didn't want me to have the lung lobe removed.

"These tests create all sorts of false alarms," he said. "You're going to be fine." But I knew he was worried about my lung lobe too, by the look in his eyes. Actually, he looked more scared than I felt, though he kept on reassuring me. "You're pregnant! Remember when we just wished for one? Now we'll have two."

This life inside me was such a vote of hope. Life had found a way to exist inside me, even though my own survival felt wobbly. I wished I could call the famous research doctor to ask her what I should do, even though I knew what she would say. Was I crazy to have this baby? I needed her help, and not in a theoretical way. Was I just being seduced by the fact that my cells could multiply in ways other than cancer? Was this too dangerous for me and for Skye?

I had a dream in which Dr. P appeared and told me exactly what to do: "Have the baby. Life is a mystery. Look at what happened to me."

I thought she had my answers. Dying of cancer felt so certain that I thought somehow my death from breast cancer was predetermined, yet now I was on a new path—growing new life inside of me. How could she have died before me, *crossing the street*?

My doctors were panicked that my tumor levels were so high, and started doing research on what could be wrong with me and where my cancer was. I was sent for an ovarian sonogram to rule out ovarian cancer because I was at such high risk after having breast cancer. When I looked at the screen, I saw the little sack of life that was there—a shadow, but not a tumor. The same doctor who had diagnosed me when I was only twenty-seven was there and knocked on the door of the examining room. "A baby? What?"

I was thirty-nine, still alive, and pregnant.

I knew that my breast cancer could *come back*, I knew that I could have a *new* breast cancer, I knew that I was at risk for *other* cancers because of my breast cancer. I also knew that I wanted a baby. I wanted to run toward life, buy rugs, and be back in the maternity ward where people sent cards of congratulation for being in the hospital. I prayed for no regrets. But even if my cancer came back, I would have a baby, and I wouldn't regret that.

My doctors kept researching the case as I waited each day, growing a baby and terrified I might also be growing a new cancer. Finally the call with the news came. "Placental growth can mimic tumor markers—you're okay."

A new life masquerading as a life-threatening situation.

My water broke on Easter Sunday. I was supposed to be at an Easter lunch at the home of my new boss. Amazingly, she was the second boss in my life whose name was Meredith, and she was a rock star too. When I checked in, the hospital was nearly deserted and the maternity ward was decorated everywhere with brightly colored cutouts of humongous eggs. It felt like a sign: My eggs had worked. And I loved being in maternity, where everyone just assumed that I was fine, and they worried about the baby. It was a personal resurrection, and my perfect little Easter bunny was wheeled in to me, in a clear glass nursery box identical to Skye's. Meredith II brought me a bedside picnic, with homemade ham and desserts. And she had big news: She had convinced Lifetime to turn my book into a movie, as part of their Stop Breast Cancer for Life campaign.

Skye wore a "Big Sister" T-shirt when we brought her baby brother home. Tyler agreed to have the circumcision done in our apartment even though he wanted it done in the hospital. His father cried during the ceremony, Tyler cried, and of course our baby boy, Hayden, cried. My dad cried; my two younger brothers kept their hands casually clasped in front of their members and looked tense. It was so emotional—there was another man joining the family. Hayden had green eyes, like my father, like my grandma Katie, who had come to this country from Poland when she was only sixteen to escape oppression for being Jewish. When I looked into Hayden's eyes, I saw my grandma's journey to America, my unlikely journeys back and forth to the same hospital for breast cancer and then babies.

I wished all my grandparents could meet the new baby, and I named Hayden for my grandpa Harry. His middle name was Connor, a nod to Tyler's Irish heritage. Hayden looked like Tyler, and seeing them together on Father's Day was a dream come true that I had never even dreamed. I got them matching orange sweaters because Tyler's favorite color was orange. It would become Hayden's favorite color.

I had to wait until after Hayden was born to check on that lung nodule again. It hadn't changed, and it never did change.

Every six months when I had it checked again in the PET scan machine, I couldn't wait to get back to my new life. I wanted to keep living outside the lines of cancer diagnoses. I had become a life *junkie*. I was hooked on things people had told me I couldn't do. Having Hayden broke the cancer sound barrier.

As soon as Hayden learned to walk, he was clomping around in Tyler's shoes, the way Skye had worn mine. Having a boy was more boisterous: Hayden would come to visit at my office, but he didn't sit and play-work like Skye; instead he'd open the drawers and throw everything on the floor. He'd want to spend an hour at the photocopying machine copying his hands. He was always on the move until one day, when he was two years old, he stopped—and started convulsing, with huge bubbles coming out of his mouth.

Hayden had had a high fever, and our babysitter, Hawa, was at home with him. I was at my office when Tyler called. "Hayden stopped breathing. He might have died! Run! Meet me at the pediatrician!" I shrieked something I don't remember and tore out of the office. I must have said "Hayden died!" to all my colleagues because they were all running after me and calling me on my cell. I was on the line with the pediatrician's office; they had called an ambulance and it was on its way to give Hayden oxygen to try to revive him.

As I rode in a taxi from my office through the park, I was crying hysterically, "Please drive faster, my son might have died. Please, hurry!" The park was bursting with life—it was June and almost every flower and tree was in bloom, taunting me with their greenness. A thought flashed into my mind: "The Lord gave, and the Lord hath taken away." There was no point in living if Hayden were dead. My life had become too big to turn back now; I couldn't give up any piece of it. I would die right then if only Hayden could live.

Living life had given me so much more to lose now.

When I burst into the pediatrician's office, Hayden was unconscious on the exam table. Hawa was near him, crying and barefoot—she had run the two city blocks from our apartment to the pediatrician's office without her shoes, carrying Hayden, wailing. The doctor was by Hayden's side, stroking his head, telling the nurse to call 911 again because the ambulance still hadn't arrived.

"Hayden!" I screamed as soon as I saw him.

The doctor looked up. "Did you see that?" Hayden had opened his eyes for a brief second. "Now that is what we call in medicine 'the maternal response.' Your boy just woke up!" He still had some bubbles around his mouth, but he stretched a little arm to touch me as the ambulance finally arrived to carry him away. I rode with him in the ambulance, to the hospital, and Tyler would meet us there.

Hawa was so thoughtful: She went home to get Hayden's beloved stuffed bunny, so when he woke up he'd have his comfort object. Hayden's Bun-Bun was a huge part of his life and so was Hawa. We had met Hawa when Skye was only three weeks old, and I was looking for a babysitter so I could go back to work right after my maternity leave. Our pediatrician had recommended Hawa: She was looking for work and he had watched with respect the way she cared for her own little boy Mohamed. It was as if Hawa had arrived on an umbrella, a Senegalese Mary Poppins to sing to my children and bring order and joy to their lives. But she hadn't really arrived so whimsically. She had come to America to find a better life and help her family back home. Her first job was bagging groceries, heading to work at four A.M.

Hayden went from being a brightly colored Easter egg to a fragile Fabergé egg. He'd had a febrile seizure, a convulsion that can be brought on by a small child's high fever, and much more common in boys than girls. The doctors at the hospital assured me that many kids are fine after a febrile seizure. And he got well and strong again, and continued to thrive until he had to interview for nursery schools in New York City.

CHAPTER 5
Joie de Vivre

*a*pplying to nursery schools in New York City is a little like applying to college, complete with essays. I was required to write a personal statement about Hayden's strengths and weaknesses and what he wanted to be when he grew up.

I had signed Skye up at a French nursery school, because Hawa spoke French. Since Hayden was a late talker, I had enrolled him in speech therapy, and I was told that speaking another language would be a disaster for him with the speech challenges he already had. So that narrowed the field of possible schools, and he had to go on interviews and staged playdates where he would be scrutinized. So did I.

"We signed you up for nursery school in a church basement," my dad said when I told him about the impending process.

"There is nothing like that in New York City," I told him.

"You're losing your grip on normalcy."

Hayden hit his New York City interviews with the strange stubborn quality that characterized his very existence. Even though every nursery school educator tried to wrangle my son, Hayden's life force could not be tamed. I wanted to explain to those teachers about the spot on my lung, and my risk in having Hayden. They didn't care—they were only assessing my son as a potential *risk* to their venerable institutions. What exactly happens in a two-year-old's interview is a closely guarded secret, but I will tell you. And I will also tell you that each interview seemed to be about finding the same thing, using different methods: a well-behaved child who followed rules.

At the first school, let's call it the "happy" school, Hayden and I went upstairs to a smallish, dark rectangular room in a church. This school's philosophy was about "play" so a collection of toys was laid out in the middle of the room, and a group of children were all allowed to "play" with the toys. Now, I am not a child psychologist, but I can tell you that most kids I know are not good at sharing toys, especially new ones. So maybe this was a subterfuge type of exercise to see how the kids negotiated the conflict of having to share those toys. But the teachers were so nice and earnest that it didn't seem like that was actually their intention.

I sensed the disaster about to strike in the room. Hayden walked right by the toys and over to a door in a wall. I had no idea where he was going but next thing I knew the lovely teacher Patty was over Hayden's shoulder. "No, Hayden. We are not opening the doors today." That was all it took for Hayden to try turning the door knob harder and harder until he gave up and noticed that right next to the door there was another door and another. Hayden had to try to open every door. Of course every door was locked, and of course every time Hayden was told not to open the door, he ignored Patty and tried to open another. Patty was so kind and gentle, putting her hand on Hayden's wrist while he was turning the knob. "Hayden. We're all playing with toys. We're not opening the doors." Hayden still tried to open every single door. I think there were twelve. By the eleventh I was about to burst out crying.

I started fantasizing about the kind of kid I wanted. The kind of kid that I would have if I were a better mother, if I had better parenting skills and DNA. I wanted a child who followed the rules. The other kids were so content playing with the toys in the middle of the room. There was a cash register with a drawer that opened, with fake money inside, and an airplane and blocks. After Hayden tried the last door, he turned and looked at me, slightly mischievous. I said, "Honey, let's go play with the toys."

I had been diagnosing Hayden with every door turn. Maybe he had ADD. Maybe he had oppositional defiant disorder. Maybe he had issues with authority. Maybe I was overreacting, but his next behavior concerned me, and no doubt Patty, even more.

Hayden lunged for the airplane that some other little boy was making go "Wheeee!" really fast. There was almost a midair collision. Patty tried to intercept Hayden and explain sharing, but Hayden took this as a reason to start pushing the cash register buttons, making the cash drawer open, while another girl already was trying to close the drawer. It was clear that Hayden couldn't share.

When I related the scene at the nursery school to Tyler, who was anxiously awaiting my call to report in, he asked, "Why couldn't you control him more?" It was tempting to blame my children's flaws on my husband, but he wanted to blame them on me.

I was dreading the next interview and I had a horrible feeling in the pit of my stomach. It should have been the dream I'd longed for: to be back in a pretty nursery school classroom with my second child. All the little chairs were arranged in a horseshoe around the teacher at story time. All the adorable little boys and girls were sitting around the circle clinging like Velcro to every word the teacher read. Lots of oohs and aahs and occasionally a sweet interruption with a very polite hand-raise to ask the teacher a question about the storyline, which demonstrated intelligence and poise. But there was an interruption. A child had dragged his chair away from the horseshoe and was standing on it, while the other kids were still straining to hear the story. The child garbled something crazy and totally indecipherable and pumped his little fist up for emphasis.

I knew that he was trying to scream "To infinity and beyond!" and channel Buzz Lightyear. Hayden was Buzz for Halloween. He was in speech therapy twice a week and it wasn't really working. Yep, that was my boy. While the other mommies congratulated their kids on how well they'd behaved at their nursery school interviews, I was left with a sense of hopelessness. I could feel myself losing my gratitude for my little miracle guy, and with it, any sense of perspective.

The next interview was even more daunting. I had lectured Hayden about not opening doors, but that was the least of my worries. The very proper headmistress greeted us in the lobby and we were put into groups of two kids (and moms). Hayden and I were assigned to a young boy with a button-down shirt *tucked in*, who *shook hands* with the headmistress. Even worse, he greeted her in Italian. "My son speaks Italian, Spanish, and French. He's a bit rusty on his English so I'll help translate if he gets confused. We are speaking Italian today." The headmistress seemed impressed. Hayden was now in speech therapy three times a week.

The headmistress went to greet Hayden with a handshake and Hayden shook! Phew! He seemed to be imitating the boy he was with, and I was so relieved. I longed for my son to be more like this boy; even a tucked-in shirt would make me so happy. When we entered the classroom, the other boy went straight to the kitchen area. He did a quick survey and started speaking rapidly in Italian to his mother. "He wants to know if there is a butter knife," his mom translated to the headmistress. "He wants to make you fresh pasta. We cook together all the time."

Mamma mia! Hayden was crashing pots and pans together and

had taken a butcher-size plastic knife and was chopping everything in sight, including the counter and the pan and his fingers. A butter knife? Next thing the other kid did was take some of the Styrofoam fruits and vegetables and arrange them in a bowl. I was sure the mommy was going to explain that they only ate organic produce, because the little boy was holding up an orange and saying something very quickly again in his perfectly accented Italian. Hayden had put completely inappropriate things into his pot to pretend-boil. One was a large fake container of orange juice.

The mommy was laughing hysterically and took the Styrofoam orange to show the teacher that Hayden had taken a real bite. "My son only drinks fresh-squeezed." The boy put away his toys and almost bowed to thank the headmistress on the way out. I was crushed.

I wanted a kid who uses a butter knife and makes me fresh pasta. I knew I could never trade Hayden—to me he was so perfect. But couldn't he just behave a little bit more?

The next interview was at a synagogue, and I was hoping my prayers would be answered in this place of worship. I was anxious, because frankly the whole interview process was dredging up something very strange inside me. I started dwelling on every interview I had ever had, and my dreams at night began with, "Tell me about yourself." I remember reading advice that if anyone asks you about a flaw, turn it into a positive. Like, "I tend to be very perfectionistic, so that can be a problem." Interviews are a lot like first dates. Fake and wrong, everyone pretending to be the best at everything and every small social interaction feeling awkward and magnified. Like the time I unwittingly wore perfume to the office of my future boss, who had an extreme migraine reaction to fragrance.

I always tried to be a pleaser in interviews and I usually succeeded. I remember one interviewer almost hired me on the spot after he asked about my waitressing experience. "The customer is always right," I said, an overt assurance that I would never challenge him if he hired me. I longed for approval, the pat on the head, the ribbon.

Again, at this synagogue interview, toys were put on a rug in the middle of the room, and this time the kids were instructed to play with those toys, which had been selected *for* them. All the other children walked over to the rug, sat down and picked a toy, and started playing. My son started scoping the joint. He walked over to a shelf in the corner of the classroom and found exactly what he was looking for: He hauled down the biggest toy he could find. It was an airplane with an entire airport, including a tower, people, and a runway. After watching Hayden drag three more oversize toys off the shelves, I sat down on one of the little wooden chairs, shaking. *Why can't he just* pretend *he's normal for these interviews?* I thought to myself, willing myself not to cry in the classroom.

I knew how wrong this was. I should see only his joie de vivre. I needed to live in the real world, which included nursery school interviews. I had to find the bridge between the mystical and the mundane. I wanted to remember the weeks of my cancer treatments when every day of living felt like a triumph and life didn't get in the way. So what if Hayden didn't get into nursery school? I should have my priorities straight.

After Ms. Weingarten at the synagogue gave me a look that seemed to say, "Didn't your mother ever teach you how to follow rules?" I tried to apologize.

"Hayden is a really good sharer. He just seems a little tired today."

"Did he miss his nap?" Ms. Weingarten was looking for a reason for this appalling behavior. I felt like she was trying to help me cheat. "We'll just let him play with the toy he's taken out," she said. "But, Hayden, it's almost time for snack. We're going to sing the cleanup song together first."

"Clean up, clean up, everybody everywhere. Clean up, clean up, everybody does his share."

I was singing the cleanup song, but Hayden wasn't. All the other kids were singing, in tune, like precious little windup robots perfectly going about the plan. As the sounds of "clean up" hung in the air, Hayden started dragging more toys to the middle of the room. He never made it to the table for snack time. Snack time unfolded in slow-motion horror. The graham crackers were distributed and every child managed to say "thank you." The kids even had napkins on their laps. They chewed with their mouths closed. They said the magic word when they wanted more juice.

"Please, Hayden! Please go have a snack! PleAaaaaaaaSe!"

The "please" I was saying was desperate, foul smelling. A beg instead of a plea. It stunk of I'm-about-to-lose-my-shit-help-me and didn't sound polite. I must have said "please" a little too rudely because a mommy in the corner stared at me. At first it was a judgment stare, like a those-shoes-don't-go-with-your-outfit stare, and I felt so embarrassed. I didn't have the wrong shoes! I had the wrong kid! I wanted the kid who was smiling back at his mommy and carefully cleaning the crumbs from his place at the table so as not to dirty the floor.

Then the mom's look became pity. She was smug, until she noticed what Hayden did next—then her look changed to shock. He ran over to the table, grabbed a graham cracker, and went back to playing with his own huge airport in the middle of the room.

The interviews continued, and my already-fragile self-esteem was about to shatter. I think it was Jackie Kennedy who said that if you bungle your kids, then you haven't done anything right. I tried to keep my game face on when Hayden went over to a dollhouse and made the people fly out the windows. First the babies flew out. "Wheeeeeee!" Hayden thought it was hilarious. Then the daddy doll flew out. Then the mommy went headfirst. If this was play therapy, then Hayden had just killed his entire family in about ten seconds. The other child playing with him said something like, "Don't make the mommy jump out the window!" And in the softest, most reassuring tone I could find, I suggested to Hayden that maybe they should just walk out the *door* instead, and I reminded him that we had window guards for babies in our apartment and people can get hurt flailing themselves out of windows. But I had lost him. It was the door! Damn it, why had I brought up the door? Hayden turned and sprinted out the door of the interview classroom. He was running down the hallway, fast, top speed, to a slide he had spied when we'd walked past another room on our way to the interview. Panting, I chased Hayden down the hall into the slide room. Hayden had climbed up and was whizzing down. "Mommy! WheeEeeeeeEeee!"

"Hayden, get off of that! We're not supposed to be in here."

The next thing I heard was screaming. The entire class had followed Hayden out of the room, Pied Piper–style. The kids were in line to get on the slide. They were screaming so loudly that other kids in other interviews heard them and ran out of their rooms and also tried to get on the slide. Hayden was a Pied Piper of pandemonium. Finally the school director ran in and blew her whistle. "Who started this? Get back to the classrooms! *Now!*"

I prayed again. This time I prayed for Hayden not to raise his hand. I had become more religious as a result of these interviews. Hayden refused to leave the slide. I finally enticed him to go back into the other classroom by suggesting that he throw more people out the window of the dollhouse. At the end of the day, on the way out of that classroom, parents were asked to sign pictures of their kids with their names, so the teachers could remember who the children were, and presumably how they behaved. I rushed by and didn't sign the photo of Hayden. Ms. Weingarten followed me into the hallway to ask if I had signed.

"I forgot to."

"Don't worry. I'll remember Hayden. *Exactly.*"

I could only imagine what her notes would say about him: Ran out of the room and caused major disruptive episode. Bad influence on otherwise orderly kids. Threw people out the window of the house.

"I'm so sorry about my son's behavior. I feel awful that I can't control him."

She gave me a sort of puzzled look.

"And my husband blames me for that. At the park Tyler looks around and sees all these well-behaved kids waiting on line for a turn at the slide. . . . When we're in restaurants Hayden is under the table, but the kid next to us has his napkin on his lap, eating his chicken nuggets with a fork and knife. . . ." I shouldn't be confessing my son's weaknesses to the woman about to evaluate his fitness for nursery school.

"Don't worry. We look for all kinds of kids to make up our classroom. Your kid . . ." She started to whisper.

Mentally I filled in the blanks: *Is an example of bad parenting. Needs Ritalin. Will never get into our school.*

She looked over at Hayden. He had taken a baby doll away from the fake washing station and was standing her under the real faucet. It looked like he was drowning the baby, holding her upside down.

"Your kid has a CEO personality."

I personally don't know any CEOs, but I remember reading lots of articles in *Fortune* magazine about the "type." I remember words like "risk taker." "Leader." "Visionary." I pictured Hayden in a tie, behind his desk, leaning back in his chair. My little Mr. CEO.

I hugged the teacher.

When the envelopes arrived, Hayden had gotten into every nursery school except one: the school where the interview had gone so well and Hayden had said "please" and "thank you." The school where the director liked him so much that she gave him a Spider-Man toy. Go figure. The school where he threw the people out the window was upset because we decided to send him somewhere else. I actually felt like I was letting them down by saying that we had selected another school.

We decided to send Hayden to the one school that spent time with the parents, not the kids. When we met with the director, she said, "Tell me about yourselves." Oh, crap, another interview. Tyler jumped in: "My wife had breast cancer." It seemed odd, because he was usually in denial about the C word, but now he was playing the Cancer Card. He knew it would work because he'd used it when we applied for our co-op, and it got us past the board.

The director leaned forward across her desk. "I like you. You've had a bump in the road."

. . . .

*H*ayden continued to have challenges: He was in speech therapy and occupational therapy, and eventually—in kindergarten—he was diagnosed with dyslexia. I found it painful that Hayden had to practice and practice the things that came so naturally to other kids. He faced rejection again in the kindergarten interview process, but by that point I was sort of over the whole thing. After one particularly bad kindergarten interview, Hayden came out and started cursing in the taxi. "Cwap! Cwap!"

"Hayden, what happened?"

"I couldn't dwaw a twiangle."

I thought about the last time I had to draw a triangle at my job. Drawing a triangle might be a bit overrated. When I opened the rejection letters, I mumbled to myself, "Your loss. My kid has a CEO personality. So what if he can't draw a twiangle." Hayden was an out-of-the-box thinker, as many dyslexics are, and they are disproportionately CEOs and entrepreneurs. That teacher had been right about my boy. Her genius was in recognizing Hayden's.

Hayden had speech therapy three times a week, and I tried to go to show support. The therapy sessions were long, and I was often asked to sit on the floor and participate.

"Hayden, we're going to practice the letter 'R.' Let's think of some things we can eat and drink that have the letter 'R,'" the therapist said.

"MaRgaRita?" Hayden looked so impressed with himself and his eyes twinkled the same way they had during his disastrous interviews. He knew that this word was not a word most kids practiced in speech therapy. He was trying to show off, despite his issues. Maybe all those nursery school interviews were cwap and Hayden was right. He had just been trying to have fun and play, and that is what two-year-olds should do.

So how did my two-and-a-half-year-old know what a margarita was? I was clearly drinking too much. I was terrified he might ask the speech therapist if she wanted sugar or salt. Before I could explain that we ate Mexican food a lot and that it was his *dad* who was the big margarita lover, his speech therapist added, "RRRRRRum."

"RRRRReally?" I cracked up.

I want normal cells in my lung and breast. But who wants a "normal" kid? Hayden was in my life to remind me to keep wonder alive. He was a gift to me, to help me always remember how sacred my present life was and always to find the joy in any situation. Hayden was pure life force, barreling at me and nursery school rules, reminding me to live harder. I would not be undone by nursery school interviews after surviving cancer. No bad interview would ever take away the joy of his life and mine.

During my cancer treatments I kept a quote from Winston Churchill near me. It was printed on a magnetized card, and it said, "Never, never, never give up." But did Winston Churchill ever worry as much as I did?

Chapter 6
How to Have a Worry-Free Day

*n*ow I have a new body part to begin worrying about after a routine scan: There is a nodule on my thyroid that they think is cancer. The word *nodule* is becoming so conversational to me since the lung nodule. I will begin to say "nodule" as often as I say a common word like "spaghetti." I speak cancer.

The doctor assures me that it is totally unrelated to my breast cancer. He has to do a biopsy immediately because the nodule looks "cold," another cancer term. But before the biopsy he needs to take about ten vials of blood. I faint from the blood draw, and then I am so dizzy that I can't stand up. The whole room is spinning, and I am in and out of consciousness. The doctor's office finally calls an ambulance to get me to a hospital for evaluation and fluids.

When the EMT comes in, puts me on a stretcher, and gets me into the ambulance, I have one simple request while we're speeding to the hospital ER. "Could you put on my lipstick?" I want my lipstick to be on when I go through the doors of Mount Sinai Hospital again.

How I enter the doors of the hospital is an important statement. I need to convince myself I will be okay even if I have cancer again.

At the hospital I am deemed okay after they give me some fluids, but I still need my nodule biopsied. I wear lipstick to my thyroid biopsy. The doctor comes at me with a humongous, knitting needle–like needle, and pushes it hard into my neck. The topical anesthetic is useless. He covers my neck wound with a large white bandage, with huge Band-Aids and surgical tape holding it in position. When I look in the mirror, I see the reality of my life in the reflection, half-bandaged but oddly glamorous and hopeful in my lipstick.

The results of the biopsy are normal, even though the doctor thought the nodule looked "cancerous and cold." The thyroid biopsy convinces me that I am not vigilant enough. The person who said it's the things you worry about that *never* happen, and the things you never worry about that *do* happen was right. I never worried about cancer before I had cancer, so I decide I need to start worrying more about everything so there is no way I could miss a possible catastrophe. I hate the feeling that one day my life is fine, and then everything could change with a needle insertion. It's the uncertainty of it all that I hate most. How will I know if it's okay to let my guard down? Cancer is like seeing a shark in the ocean: After that, fins will seem to appear everywhere. Is it a sore throat, or cancer? Pulled muscle, or cancer? Flu, or cancer?

As long as I can remember, I have worried. I thought that having cancer would somehow cure me of worrying because it would trump every other worry. It even became my mantra to keep me from worrying about the mundane: Don't worry, it's not cancer. But instead I *still* find that even trivial worries are worthy of worry because if I stopped worrying about the trivial, I'd worry that it meant I was disengaging from my life. I decide that I need to be even more vigilant.

Being a mom has given me an entire new genre of things to worry about. There was the day that Hayden woke up with gigantic balls. We went to the ER, and he was diagnosed with epididymitis, which meant that the lining of his testicles was swollen. So I have to add epididymitis to my list of worries. I am worried that my current list of worries is both too long and might not be complete:

- I was worried that I would never be able to get pregnant. But now I worry about my kids taking the SAT, not being happy, getting bizarre conditions (like swollen balls) that I don't even know the name of.
- I'm worried my kids have too much homework.
- I'm worried my daughter's boyfriend will break her heart even though she doesn't have a boyfriend yet.
- I worry about the future, but in the same breath I worry there won't be a future.
- I'm worried that I haven't enjoyed the present because I'm worried about the future.
- I'm worried that if the cancer comes back I won't be okay.
- I'm worried that I haven't made the most of my life even though the cancer hasn't come back.
- I'm worried that if I live more, I will keep falling more in love with life . . . and then I will have more to lose if my cancer comes back.
- I'm worried that if I give up my worry, I don't know what will replace it.
- I'm worried that I don't drink enough green juice and eat organic.
- I'm worried Skye thinks I am not cool. I'm worried I gave her a defective gene.
- I'm worried I'm not nice enough to my mom . . . still.

- I'm worried that I don't like shopping as much anymore. Does that mean I'm losing my zest for life?
- I'm worried that cancer hasn't given my life enough gravitas.
- I'm worried that I should know better than anyone that life is short and brief and it is important not to worry and just enjoy it and be in the moment and be happy.
- I'm worried every time I have a headache: It might be a brain tumor.

I have tried to relax or even "chillax" as Skye suggested. My parents have meditated all their lives, but I'm too high-strung to meditate. I spend my entire meditation worrying that I am not relaxing enough. But I *am* open to new relaxation methods: My heart has started racing and I am worried, so Tyler thinks I should try acupuncture. He schedules an appointment with Dr. Cai, an acupuncturist.

When I meet Dr. Cai I sense this man might hold a very strange key to quelling my worry. After a quick examination to determine my energy flow, life force, or chi, he sums up my entire life story. "Traffic congestion is going wrong way" is how he describes it. He puts needles in me, and tells me to "breathe and relax." And I do feel relaxed, but then I start to worry about all the needles in my body. They remind me of the needles from IVs, from chemo shots. I really like Dr. Cai, but before every visit I worry too much about the stabs of the little needles.

I've been in therapy my whole life, and it hasn't really stopped the worrying, but it has made me more *aware* of it and what a burden it is. My cancer therapist, Dr. Haber, assures me that sometimes there are no reasons for life's tragedies: "Geralyn, sometimes things are unknowable. Like why you got cancer." But she also says, "Why look for clouds on a sunny day?" And she suggests a little bit of medication too.

My psychiatrist, a.k.a. "Try Not to Worry So Much" Dr. Goodman (that really is his name), believes that I can worry less. He has even set a goal for me: I should try to have a worry-free day. "Wouldn't it be nice for you to have a worry-free day and just relax and be fine with that?"

"Okay," I tell him in all seriousness, "I'll make a list of all the things I need to *not* worry about to have a worry-free day."

He laughs. "That isn't what I was expecting."

When he speaks with me, Dr. Goodman always finds a way to find something positive about what I'm worrying about. It is a rare gift. And he seems impressed with my progress. We kept discovering good things that I hadn't thought could ever happen to me, but they did.

"You were worried you wouldn't have a baby because of your cancer, and now you have two. You were worried you wouldn't live, and you did." He also writes me a prescription for Klonopin, which *really* helps with the worrying.

When I take my first Klonopin, it's like I *can't* worry anymore. It is the weirdest feeling. I think I should be worrying that I can't worry anymore . . . but finally, I'm not.

After I google how Klonopin actually works, I feel a bit less worried. Wikipedia tells me:

Clonazepam acts by binding to the benzodiazepine site of the GABA receptors, which enhances the electric effect of GABA binding on neurons, resulting in an increased influx of chloride ions into the neurons. This further results in an inhibition of synaptic transmission across the central nervous system.

Yeah, baby! Bring on that inhibition of synaptic transmission across my central nervous system. Oooooh. That feels so good! It is sort of awesome but terrifying. If Klonopin makes me less worried, I'll be less vigilant, and if I'm less vigilant, how will I be safe? How can I let my army/navy/air force/marine guard down about cancer, about life in that ambiguous world?

The K helps so much that I start to worry about what I would do without it. I worry that I might become addicted to something that makes me feel so calm. I worry I could never not worry without the drug. And then I feel gratitude that a doctor has clearly worried enough to invent an anti-worry drug.

I have read some self-help books about being in the moment, the "now," and just appreciating the present tense. I find a quote I love: Mother Teresa says, "Be happy in the moment, that's enough. Each moment is all we need, not more."

But every time I am in that moment, I need to know there is a next one coming. How can I feel the moment is enough? I just want to know my ending, know the cancer won't be back, and know that I am okay. I want to know that I lived "happily ever after" like a fairy tale. My brother counsels me, "Don't future-trip." I love to make up endings to all my problems, which involve doom and strange and awful events.

And then, something more surreal and horrible than I could make up: Hawa has a sore throat that isn't getting better. We were worried she had the flu, that she needed antibiotics. But she is diagnosed with stage 4 cancer, a head and neck tumor. It also seemed insane that I finally got to have my miracle children, met this kind and wise woman who would always be there for my kids if I got sick again, and now she might be taken away because of cancer. She was the one who was supposed to be a stable presence for my kids. I remember when my mom and I interviewed Hawa. I remember what she looked like when she first held Skye. I knew they fit together.

Hawa knew all the answers I didn't about how to raise kids. Like when we were at the pediatrician with Skye when she had to get four vaccinations in one day. I was panicked.

"Hawa, I don't think I should stay in the room, because Skye will think that I'm letting someone hurt her. I'll wait outside."

"No, Mommy!"

Hawa called me "Mommy" and I called her "Mommy #2."

"Mommy, stay in the room. Skye needs to know that whatever happens to her, you are there for her."

I entered the doctor's exam room and cradled my daughter on my lap as she screamed with each successive needle that was jabbed into her fleshy little arm. Hawa held my hand as I held Skye's, and she squeezed my hand so tight, it distracted me from Skye's wailing. Telling me to stay in the room was the right advice. I was there for my daughter.

And now it is I who has to go into the room and squeeze Hawa's hand. She has been admitted to Mount Sinai Hospital for her neck biopsy, a surgical procedure. I hear her moaning in the recovery room. I want to be with Hawa when the resident goes in to give her the bad news. And I'll also have to tell the same news to her family, who have flown in from Africa. They have looked so worried, waiting all day in the family lounge, speaking French with each other. Every time I go to check on them they stand to greet me, with such anxious eyes.

I wait for the doctor in the hall outside the recovery room, and beg her to explain to Hawa that she has cancer, but that they can cure her.

The resident, holding her clipboard, annoyed, is having none of it. "I can't say that. It might not be true." She refuses to say the word "cure" when she reports the diagnosis.

I want the doctor to be hopeful. Maybe it is unreasonable for me to ask that, but I want to give Hawa hope. I remember when my doctor had told me my own cancer news: "You do have breast cancer. But we are going to cure you." I had never heard the words "cancer" and "cure" together before.

"I can't promise that." The resident is shaking her head and staring at her clipboard, deliberately not making eye contact with me. There is no way I can get her to budge.

"Please just be really nice. Tell her there's hope. Tell her it will be okay. Please!"

The resident is shaking her head harder. She won't budge.

"Okay, can *I* tell her that she has cancer? I'm a survivor. I can relate to her. Let me deliver the news. I know how to handle this. Clearly you're not being as sensitive as I think you should be. There's a woman moaning and crying in there; she's already in pain from her surgery."

"Hospital regulations require that I tell the patient."

I am about to freak out on this robotic resident.

"Would it *kill you* to be nice to her? She has cancer!"

The resident turns her back on me and marches into the room. I trail behind her and give her the evil eye when she is telling Hawa, "You have cancer, Ms. Kane."

She turns to leave, and I body-block her.

"Don't you also want to tell Hawa about how she's going to start her treatment soon and it will be okay? . . . You know, how good the treatment can be . . ."

The doctor sidesteps me and leaves the room.

I climb into Hawa's bed and squeeze her hand. She is wailing, like Skye did from her vaccinations.

"Hawa, look at me. I am okay. You will be too. I promise. I'm going to take care of you the way you've taken care of me and the kids. Hawa, God meant for us to be together. You've been my guardian angel; I'm going to be yours."

I bring her some water because her mouth is so dry from anesthesia. I help her take a sip, and I remember her teaching Skye how to drink from the Big Girl glass and not use the sippy cup. Hawa is so uncomfortable from the pain, and she is crying again. I ask the nurse for liquid Tylenol, like Hawa has given to my kids when they've had pain. I also ask for a Klonopin, but the nurse rebuffs me. That has to be ordered by a physician in psychiatry. Hawa is sweating and I give her a little sponge bath, like she has done for Skye and Hayden hundreds of time before bed. I tuck her into her hospital bed and kiss her forehead. I need to go tell her family the diagnosis.

"I promise you, we are going to beat this, Hawa."

I used to hate it when people told me that. Am I being a hypocrite now?

As I leave Hawa's room and walk through the hallway, I stumble to the window and hold on to the ledge for support. The hallway is spinning, and I am flooded with the same sensations I had when I was first diagnosed. I feel all hope draining out of me as I look outside the hospital window, sentenced again to the cancer ward. I see the automatic sliding doors opening and closing in front of the emergency-room entrance to the hospital. Hawa and I are somehow trapped together in this hospital, on the same side now, unable to leave. This is our world now; we are on the cancer side. The other side—the normal side—is a world we can visit, but then we must return to the cancer side, where we belong.

When I get to the lounge and tell Hawa's family, there is so much crying and speaking in French. The word "cancer" sounds so much more elegant with a French accent, but just as deadly.

"J'ai eu un cancer."

I had done a quick google so I could remind them in French that I had had it too. We all hug. I promise them that Tyler and I will take care of Hawa and get her the best medical care. Tyler and I call doctors and review all the medical literature.

Tyler cries when he sees how dire her prognosis is.

We spend hours on Medline and the Internet and find a clinical trial for Hawa that is high-dose chemo and radiation, created by a German doctor. He is now in Chicago; we get him on the phone, and he explains there is a clinical trial in New York City that we can try to get her into. It is a barbaric treatment of both chemo and radiation, together, in high doses to increase the effectiveness of the toxicity. But it will spare her surgery that would remove her voice box and disfigure her face. In the past, patients like Hawa—if they had their voice boxes removed—had to learn to speak with an artificial voice box. The thought of not having Hawa's singsong French-accented voice in her son's life, in my family's life, is not an option.

I need to be even stronger for Hawa than I remember being for myself. I have to believe that she can be cured, that she'll live, even though I am not so sure I will. Hawa is my Senegalese sister. We somehow found each other in this world. I always thought she would be there for my children if I died, but now I tell her that I will be there for her son, Mohamed, if she dies. She has taken care of my children; now it is time for us to take care of her.

My visits to Dr. Goodman sustain me. He reminds me, "It makes sense that you're worried about Hawa, but try to remind yourself that you survived and there's every reason to think she will too. Try to relax." He tells me that I have something called "anticipatory anxiety" in addition to the garden variety of worrying, which means that I worry about worrying about things. I see it as an opportunity to take more Klonopin.

I think about the idea that the things we *don't* worry about can happen—random types of disasters can sneak up on us. How crazy-making that is.

I'm back in the white hallways of the hospital with Hawa during her treatment. There is one day when her neck is burned very badly from the radiation, and she is whispering to me how much everything hurts. She tells me they are coming to get her to wheel her in for more radiation and she doesn't want to go.

"Please, Gerrraline. Please, don't let them take me."

I ask her doctors to wait and let her rest a bit, and I run home to my apartment to get one of my favorite hats, which someone gave me when I was bald—a bright pink cowboy hat. I never could truly pull it off, but I knew that Hawa would rock it with her dark black, almost purple skin.

I arrive at the hospital out of breath just as they are wheeling Hawa down the hall to the radiation suite. I show her the hat. She starts to laugh, then cry, then laugh again.

"Only for you, Mommy!"

"Ms. Hawa, we *love* your hat! *Wow!*" All the technicians have stopped wheeling Hawa to admire her.

I was not going to let my Senegalese sister go. I was going to fight as hard for her life as she had for mine. My kids never had to see me sick, but they did see Hawa in the hospital. Hayden just jumped into her bed and wouldn't leave. I had to pull him off crying when visiting hours were over. Skye made her get-well cards, and she worried and cried a lot about Hawa. One day, the school nurse called sounding very upset: "Mrs. Lucas, Skye has a sore throat. She thinks she has cancer."

I bought a wig for Hawa to wear for her son and my kids because she didn't want them to be upset or scared when they first had to see her completely bald. She had been wearing scarves and the pink cowboy hat, but now there was nothing left on her head.

When Skye saw Hawa in the wig, she asked her to take it off so she could see her without it. Hawa was reluctant.

"I like you better bald, Hawa," Skye said. "You shine now."

· · · ·

As I am trying not to worry so much about my Senegalese sister, an invitation arrives for me from my other unofficial "sisters": the Zeta Tau Alpha sorority. I have been working on breast cancer awareness campaigns across the country with the Zetas on sorority campuses, because breast cancer is their national philanthropy. They would like to officially initiate me as an honorary member of the Zeta Tau Alpha sorority because of the work I am doing to educate young women about breast cancer. When I was growing up, I had always wanted a sister. I had two younger brothers I loved, but there was something about having a sister, like Hawa.

For my initiation I had to wear an all-white outfit—dress, sweater, and shoes. White always scared me—white bandages, white sheets, white hallways—but now white was sorority whites. They walked me into a special room, but I can't reveal what happened in there because I am a sister now and sworn to secrecy. The room was dark and there were women's voices, and I cried after the ceremony, standing before my five hundred new sisters, all wearing white for me.

I was an about-to-turn-thirty-nine-year-old sorority sister!

The Law of the Unexpected must apply to happiness too.

CHAPTER 7
Deathbed Regrets

*W*atching Hawa in the cancer ward made me think about what had happened since I had left the cancer ward. I had finally had my miracle kids, but I wasn't spending any time with them. I was either on a conference call, in a meeting, on my way to work, or e-mailing work from home.

The problem was that I was *madly* in love with my job. It was the in-love, romantic phase of love, where I couldn't bear to be away from it for a single moment. I was so smitten with my job that my family was jealous. When I was with one, the other always seemed to want or need me *right now*.

I should have remembered the wisdom from oncology nurses I met when I was invited to speak at the meeting of the Oncology Nursing Society. These women and men see death a lot and they are my true heroes. I interviewed a few before my speech.

"How do you do it?"

Oncology nurse: "We drink. A lot." Then, tears.

"Every patient has taught me something."

"Everyone seems, at the end, to wish they'd worked less, and spent more time with family and friends."

The old cliché is that no one on her deathbed wishes she'd spent more time working.

But my cancer had made me work harder. When I was at *20/20* and having chemo, I got promoted. During treatment, I worried about work, not cancer cells. I loved TV: It was so amazing to put something out into the world in that way. It was my responsibility to find story ideas for the show, so I got to work on all kinds of pieces: from the serious—we were the first network to report on honor killings of Jordanian women—to the provocative, about a woman who had seventeen plastic surgeries to become a human Barbie doll. I also got to work on stories I discovered as an insider in the cancer community, like the story about women who *didn't* have breast cancer but decided to remove their healthy breasts and ovaries to avoid *getting* cancer—long before the discovery of the breast cancer gene.

I was worried I might be considered damaged goods and be denied a job because I was a cancer survivor. My brothers, both attorneys, told me that would be illegal, but I was worried about perception. Would employers be worried about taking a chance on me if I could die soon?

I decided to put my cancer information on my resume under the "Awards" section: *Self* magazine had given me an award for my cancer activism. Cancer was a strange credential, but I was determined to use what I had.

I was hired at Lifetime Television to work in programming, but I took the job because of their breast cancer campaign, which was the brainchild of Meredith II. I got to produce celebrity biographies. I worked on the bio of former first lady Laura Bush, and that took me to the White House. I told the story of Elizabeth Taylor's great loves and great jewels. My favorite profile was about fashion designer Betsey Johnson, which I did for the Stop Breast Cancer for Life campaign.

Betsey became a friend and launched my first book in all of her stores. She created a special Big Lips T-shirt (I wore it for my book jacket photo), and she sold the tees to raise funds for breast cancer research. After the profile of Betsey, my dream came true and I was transferred full-time to Meredith's team to work on other issues important to women, like ending violence against women, breast cancer awareness, and encouraging women to vote and run for elected office. What I loved about that job was that it was advocacy embedded in programming.

Skye had some amazing perks because of my job. I thought she'd be impressed that I was sitting in the front row at the Betsey Johnson fashion show during Fashion Week in New York. There were other projects with Christina Aguilera, Taylor Swift, Nicole Kidman. But the celebrities didn't impress Skye; she just wanted me home with her.

I brought Skye to the LA party and premiere of the TV movie made from my own book, *Why I Wore Lipstick to My Mastectomy*. It was at a very chic club (Justin Timberlake was launching his own clothing line that night in the same club) and was so Hollywood, very dark and oozing cool. The entire cast of *Scrubs* was there because Sarah Chalke was playing *me*! I sat next to Zach Braff, and Skye walked the red carpet with me. We posed for photos and I thought, *Wow, I can have it all.*

Until the movie was over and the lights went up in the club.

Skye had fallen asleep—the time difference was too hard for her: She was only six. "Mommy, I want to go! I'm *tired*!"

"But, Skye, there's an after-party."

People were crowding around me, and Skye started to cry. I was being pulled in all directions—celebrated in the room, but a huge disappointment to my daughter.

"Mommy, I want to go! *Now!*"

But everyone was headed to the after-party for the movie about *me*—so it would have been really bad form to skip it. The director of the movie had a little boy Skye's age, and he and his wife spotted Skye crying. They offered to take her home with them.

Skye glared at me and continued crying. "Who's more important to you, Mommy? Your own daughter, or all these people you don't know?"

I couldn't answer her question. The director and his wife pried a shrieking Skye away from me.

There were other glamorous job moments that I thought would be amazing Mommy-and-Me memories for Skye, but they sometimes turned sour. I took my mother and eight-year-old Skye with me to Japan to launch my book there. The plan was that she and Mom would fly home before me, because I had to give a speech at a medical school outside of Tokyo. It would have meant too much travel for Skye, and she'd have been bored at the hospital in a room full of grown-ups speaking Japanese. But when it came time for them to go—even though I had talked Skye through all the mechanics of the trip—she began to sob that she didn't want to leave me.

We were at a mall in Tokyo, and it was pouring rain. I walked my mom and Skye out to the waiting taxi and hugged them good-bye. Skye wouldn't let me go, and finally my mother had to pull my daughter away. I think I cried more than Skye as I made my way back to the hotel. I didn't want to be saying good-bye to her all the time because I was working so much. On the other hand, sometimes I cried because I was so happy to be *away* from my kids, and Tyler too. There was nothing like having a big bed, a remote, and a bathroom all to myself on a business trip.

One morning, as I was in a cab rushing to my office for a huge meeting, my cell phone started ringing: It was my daughter's school, the nurse's office. I couldn't screen. I had to answer.

"Mrs. Lucas, Skye has lice. A very bad case. Nits, live ones . . . Please come get her immediately." Just as the school nurse was finishing her sentence, call-waiting was showing me that my office was ringing too. A colleague. Call-waiting was such a concrete reminder of the two worlds I straddled: work and home. I asked the nurse to please hold, sorry, and clicked over.

"The celebrity we're shooting is asking for a hair-and-makeup allowance of five thousand dollars. We don't have it in our budget. You have to negotiate it down." As we discussed strategy, I totally forgot that the nurse was on the other line. Suddenly I remembered. I quickly wrapped up with the boss and clicked back to lice.

"Mrs. Lucas, you should probably hire Licenders to come delouse your home too, so she doesn't get re-infested."

The irony of the situation wasn't lost on me: There were hair problems on both calls—if only I could have done a conference call with both parties and found a solution. I was tempted to ask the celebrity hair-and-makeup people demanding so much money if they would throw in a delousing for their price and we could call it a day. It was close to impossible to bring these two distant worlds together: the glamorous TV job I worked at and my constantly morphing family life.

I diverted the taxi to my daughter's school, and when I arrived in the nurse's office, I saw a woman in a white coat examining a redhead's braided hair, under a super-bright white light, using a magnifier. Her hands were gloved and she was carefully inspecting the part between the braids. Skye was huddled in the corner with a group that seemed to have LOUSERS stamped on them. Every once in a while there was an anxious itch in the room, loud in the silence. A sound like sandpaper doing its job. I started to itch too, just from being there. My daughter's face was like an Etch A Sketch toy—at first flushed with a huge *relief* to see me; then the relief completely disappeared and became *upset* as she blurted, "Mom, what took you so long to get here?" Then the Etch A Sketch knobs turned and landed on a final expression: She was looking at my shoes. "Why are you wearing *those* with that dress?" (I was wearing Uggs with a dress to give my feet a rest because I was going to be in stilettos all night at a fund-raiser for the American Cancer Society.)

"Mommy is Dream Girl tonight. Did you forget, sweetie?" The words "Dream Girl" hung in the air and smelled suspicious, as if I were the furthest thing from a dream to the daughter I had so disappointed by working instead of being there for every moment of her life. The evidence against me was overwhelming.

Like the time she literally took her first steps in a Stride Rite shoe store on Eighty-Third and Third Avenue while I was on a conference call across town. Hawa called me crying, she was so excited. The entire store was cheering, even the jaded shoe guy who must have handled eight hundred toes in kids' shoes while explaining to each uptight mom that the shoes were indeed big enough; the child had room to grow. He got to see my daughter's first steps and I didn't. "Your baby girl walked!" Hawa was telling me on my cell over the cheering in the background, while I had muted the conference call I was supposed to be on. I heard the joy I was not part of. It was as if she had taken first steps on the moon, the cheers were so loud. I needed to get back to the conference call. I had been on mute too long and it was probably my turn to talk. The Halloween costumes, the playdates, the sick days. I wanted to take her to the pediatrician when she was sick. I wanted to pick her up at school and have her run into my arms and scream, "Mommy's here!" I wanted to be in two places at once so badly.

But there in the nurse's office, I wished I could be at the celebrity photo shoot where there were no lice. I was trying to copy down the nurse's information about Licenders, but I had a call coming in from my boss. Lice or boss? Boss or lice? I held up one finger to the nurse, and my daughter's eyes widened. What could be more important now than her delousing?

Meredith's voice sounded weird and mine must have too: "Hey, I'm in a meeting. . . . Could I call you right back?" (Well, it was sort of a meeting. With the nurse. About lice.)

"It's urgent. We have to talk. How long will it be?" I had never heard Meredith speak like this.

"Soon, I promise. I'll call you back soon."

It sounded like I was about to get fired, but first I needed to de-louse my daughter. My priorities felt okay for once. My daughter grabbed me. "Mom. We have to go. *Now.*" My daughter's classmates had started to pile into the hall between classes and now word would be out about her lice. As I turned to leave, I saw the light reflecting off the magnifying glass the nurse was using to examine the girls' scalps for lice. It was huge and it could reveal even the tiniest nits that would hatch and become lice. I asked her if she could check my scalp to see if I was infected too, because now I couldn't stop itching. As she was looking, examining, I pictured my life being under that magnifier and I wondered if the nurse could see the choices I had made. My daughter's ballet recital, at which I spent the whole time texting with the office. Her birthday, where I struggled to stay awake because I had taken the red-eye home from another business trip. I was so tired, it hurt to sing "Happy Birthday." The apple-picking field trip, where I couldn't ride the tractor because there was no cell signal and I had another conference call.

Miraculously the nurse couldn't see any larvae on my scalp.

"Mom, hurry up!" My daughter caught me spacing out. The nurse explained that the minute we got home we had to call Licenders, and put all Skye's stuffed animals into plastic bags to suffocate any lice, and wash all the sheets in boiling-hot water to kill the nits. My phone was ringing again, vibrating actually. There were no cell calls allowed in her school.

Meredith. I screened her because I needed to call Licenders. It was a more crucial decision than I realized: It turned out that I had a lurk-ing case of lice, imperceptible even under the magnifier. I was infected too. The nits were a symbol, I would later decide. My problems strad-dling work and home were about to hatch if I didn't deal with them in an extreme way. I needed a magnifier, fine-tooth comb, some intense rinse, to clean up my life.

I panicked when I realized that I had hair-and-makeup people coming to *my apartment too*, at noon, to make me look like a Dream Girl for the fund-raiser that night. And my mom was coming in to see me win that award for my cancer work. I needed my mommy. On the way home we had to stop at the drugstore for an anti-lice shampoo called Kwell, which smelled like furniture polish. Was it safe to put that so close to our brain cells?

My mom arrived just in time for me to start pushing her around. I was trying to be nicer to her, but I had lapses. "Put all Skye's stuffed animals in a plastic bag, put this stuff on her hair, call Licenders. I need to call my boss." I was being obnoxious to my poor mom, who'd been hit with this lice tsunami.

"Your boss can wait." My mom looked at me like I had all my priorities wrong, and I sort of knew it, but I needed to call my boss. So I called my boss even though my mom was glaring at me.

"Pour yourself a glass of wine." I did what she told me to, because I did love and respect her. "Our department is being transferred to LA. We want you to come with us. Would you consider moving your family to LA? Think about it. This is a shock to all of us. I'm so sorry, I'm so disappointed too."

Meredith must have poured herself a glass of wine before she had to deliver the news. I knew I'd miss the glasses of wine we'd shared after big launches.

The thought of my job, wearing sunglasses, taking meetings, made me nauseated. *My* job would go on without *me* and become an LA player. It seemed so unfair. I said to Meredith, "Okay, let me think about this."

As I hung up the phone, I gulped down the drink I had poured and started to cry. Not because I was losing my job, the job I had chosen over my daughter so many times, but because I'd been so mean to my mom when she walked into my apartment to be here for me to-night. *She* deserved the award. She had come to every chemo; she'd been at my bedside. She had cleaned up my vomit and I had just given her a verbal vomit. Why was I so mean to my mom? Especially when things were going wrong in my life and she was trying to help?

I needed to get *one thousand dollars* from the cash machine to pay Licenders. I thought about what I could do with all that money. Then I thought about all the conference calls I needed to do to afford to de-louse my daughter. But now they were going away. What would I do without those conference calls? Whom would I talk to?

I told my mom my job was gone and I was panicking. My mom got angry.

"After all you gave to that corporation, your job went away in three minutes. Well, your daughter needs you now. You have two years left where she'll actually want to be with you. Then she's gone. She'll come back, but it will be a long, long time. . . ." Mom looked wistful, as if she might cry, and she knew exactly what she was talking about.

"You won't get this chance again. Trust me. I still drive by the school bus stop wishing you were there. I would give anything to be there for you now."

But she was here for me *now*. My mom worked when I was little. She brought home the bacon and tried to fry it up in a pan. She had three kids in less than four years, and we were all in diapers at the same point and she was tired all the time. She worked in an elementary school as a school guidance counselor, helping other kids, but she missed her own. She had to work; I've had to work.

She told me that she'd get the cash for the Licender lady; she packed up the stuffed animals in plastic bags, stripped the bed, threw all the sheets in the washing machine, and made lunch for my daughter. I needed her today maybe more than I did then.

When Licenders arrived, my daughter announced that she would get the door. We had rehearsed what she should say because I didn't want the fancy hair-and-makeup people to know that she had lice. "*Maman*, my French tutor is here!"

As I was leaving for the Dream Girl Ball that night, my daughter stopped me in the hallway, studying me. I imagined she wanted to tell me how surprisingly good I looked, or maybe that she was proud that I was getting an award from the American Cancer Society for my work helping cancer patients.

"Mom, I don't know how to say this to you. . . ." Maybe she was happy that my job was moving so we could spend more time together bonding?

"*Don't* walk out the door. Your butt looks so big in that skirt. Change. Seriously, look in the mirror! No one else will tell you the truth, except me, your daughter!"

I walked off the stage backward that night, just in case my daughter was right, which was pretty tricky in my super-high heels. That night was the last time I would wear heels in a long time because my transition to full-time momminess didn't involve many high heels. I decided the best way to separate from my job was to rip it off, like a Band-Aid. I was going to do a cannonball into the mommy pool. I didn't want to start looking for a new job right away. It would be like having a Bloody Mary to cure a hangover. I needed to try to be more of a mom, and really try to be more "there" for my kids. A new job would mean working even longer hours and expending even more energy to impress a new boss.

I'd have a bit of severance from my old job, and we'd scale way back. And there would be new expenses for our family: I had always provided the health insurance through my corporate job. Even though he was a doctor, Tyler had to pay so much more for our health insurance through his job than mine. He was a bit surprised at how much more it would cost him to pay for the things that had been my contributions to the family, but he was supportive anyway, now that I wanted to spend more time with the kids. Tyler and I had always tried to support each other's careers. I wasn't saving lives at work, but I loved my job as a TV journalist. I loved my job so much that when Tyler had to do specialized training in Philadelphia, I took a train to and from New York City every day to keep working. I had showed up for work every day during chemo.

I'd been working since I was eleven years old. I'd been a babysitter, a busgirl, a waitress, a lifeguard, a swim instructor, a camp counselor, a retail salesgirl, a marketing executive, an intern at a TV station, a TV producer, a writer, a speaker. I always put on my identity with each of these jobs, like putting on my coat in the morning. The jobs made me feel purposeful, like I was contributing something to someone. Now that Lifetime had left me, I was about to start at the hardest job of my life: full-time mom.

I thought it would be so cool to finally have the opportunity to drop Hayden off at his little preschool program. Before, when I went to a job, I'd never had the chance to do drop-off or pickup. I felt so responsible, like a mom with a capital *M*, the first time I breezed through the school door. Hayden waved to the security guards and I continued to smile until they stopped me and asked for ID. "I'm his mom," I said sort of smugly.

"You are not in the system." The guard frowned back, and I humbled myself and registered. That should have been a sign to me that maybe I didn't belong, but I persisted. When I kissed Hayden goodbye at the classroom after actually meeting his teachers for the first time, Hayden threw himself on the floor and started to scream.

"Don't go, Mommy!" He screamed so loudly that all the other moms peeked their heads outside of their classrooms to catch the show.

"Why don't you stay for a bit; he's probably anxious because you haven't dropped him off before," his teacher, Lisa, sweetly offered.

A bit turned into three weeks.

My new office: a kiddy classroom desk at Hayden's preschool, with a small chair that I was so uncomfy in. I was being instructed on how to make something out of Floam. Floam is the new Play-Doh, but it is sort of Styrofoamish and comes in neon colors. It feels smooth and cool, and doesn't get hard like Play-Doh. Every once in a while, Lisa came over to me to give me some help with my Floam technique. And thank goodness it was snack time soon because I was starving. I wished they served coffee at snack time because I had skipped my coffee to drop off Hayden, and I had a pounding caffeine-withdrawal headache, but Hayden still wouldn't let me leave him. Every day I made intricate Floam creations, as if taking out all my work experience on the poor Floam, and I started bringing coffee for snack time. I even raised my hand to share at circle time. It was sort of awesome.

This was my new normal, and I slowly started to adjust to my new "office" with Hayden. There was something really cool about sitting in a circle every day and being assigned a task, like cleaning up after a snack. My favorite job was wiping down the tables because I got to use this little squirt bottle.

I felt bad when some of the other kids in the classroom started getting separation anxiety because I was in the classroom. The teacher explained to me that most of the kids in the class had already separated from their babysitters and parents, a gradual and arduous process that had started back in September. But I arrived in January, when almost everyone had settled in. I was separating from my job, so I had sympathy for separation, such a painful exercise. Whenever a kid cried about missing her mom, I wanted to cry and nod about missing my job.

Hayden introduced me to his friend Joseph, a too-handsome-to-be-only-three-years-old Italian boy wearing a gold charm around his little neck.

"You have such beautiful hands, Hayden's mommy."

I felt sort of hot when I played with my Floam because Joseph kept staring at my hands. So inappropriate, but I needed a bit of attention. No one had ever told me I had beautiful hands! When I kneaded the Floam, I added extra flourish, just for Joseph. When I saw him staring at my hands, it gave me a little rush. I was a hand hottie. But I tried not to get too conceited. Maybe he just missed his mommy.

I missed getting dressed in the morning like I had somewhere important to go. These days I was in a ponytail and sweats. In my former working life, the purpose of my high heels was always, I thought, to look great in the boardroom, but probably they were more of a signal that I didn't belong on the playground. I missed having a lockable door so badly that often I locked myself in our bathroom at home just to remember the feeling of being in a place where no one could disturb me.

I missed the office most when my daughter shut her bedroom door on me after I'd waited all day for her to come home so I could finally see her. She was behind closed doors, and I wasn't invited. I wondered if I had already missed that magic window with Skye, the one that my mom had warned me about. Skye was getting older and it seemed like she needed me less.

I missed going to meetings in the corporate boardroom and actually having people listen to my ideas as if I had something to contribute. I felt lonely—I didn't have my water-cooler friends to gossip with and feel validated by.

I missed the business trips where I had too many places to go and not enough hours for all the people I needed to see. I even missed the long, long conference calls. Sometimes. These days my calls were with teachers, dance instructors, and tutors, and my kids always interrupted me when I was talking on the phone. I had always been judgmental of moms who let their kids interrupt them when they were on the phone. I'd never do that, I had promised myself. Now, whatever conversations I had included sidebars with Hayden and Skye. I guess that qualified as conference calls, sort of.

Somehow I never had the time to take the morning shower I'd thought I would take three days ago. My hygiene had become what my son's was. When I begged him to take a shower, he replied, "I can't really smell myself." I got it: If I don't smell, I don't shower. I used to wear fabulous perfumes called Love in White and Love in Black. I used to alternate my fragrances, and I smelled so good that people would swoon, "Mmm, what are you wearing?"

As a full-time mom, most days I smelled like McDonald's. My toes used to be pedicured; now they were shoved into sneakers. When I grabbed my sneakers from the closet, I caught a glimpse of the heels I used to wear. They seemed so lonely, sitting on the shelf with no-where to go. My heels and I should have had a glass of wine and dis-cussed our lives. They must have been mad at me because I had moved on to sneakers. Like spurned lovers, those heels appeared to be mop-ing. What wouldn't I have given to be complaining that my heels were pinching my toes again?

There was a time when I had standards for my appearance, and they weren't even that high. I had loved wearing black suits with black tights to work, and I'd had my hair blown out regularly. I'd always done my makeup in the cab, going to my job, and I'd always worn bright red lipstick. My standards were slipping and Hawa had no-ticed. She seemed quite concerned about my appearance these days—she even stopped me from leaving the house.

"Where are your earrings? Where is your makeup? You know my rule that you are not allowed to leave the house in sweatpants anymore."

I missed the office routine and how productive I'd felt. The min-utes at home frittered into hours, the hours piled up into dinnertime, and my watch felt as if it had melted. The worst part of my new mommy job was when Tyler came home from his office and asked with a mixture of curiosity and voyeurism, "What did you do all day?" I didn't know what to say, but I must have been doing something because I was sticky all the time now, usually from something being wiped on me, or from wiping my hands on myself because something gross that should have been thrown away had ended up in my hands instead.

"Mom, are you the garbage?" Hayden asked me in all seriousness one day at pickup from preschool.

"Yeah, I guess so." I didn't know whether to laugh or cry. He spit out whatever was in his mouth—sticky but sweet-smelling—into my open hand. And to prove that I *was* his garbage, he wiped his sticky hand on my jeans, leaving a gooey trail. Another mom, also waiting in the hallway, noticed and offered me a wipe. Her son had just done the same thing to her. We really hit it off: Her son had also thrown himself down screaming the first time she'd dropped him off. The conversation was going amazingly well until she said, "Do you have a card?"

She wanted to make a plan to hang out, and all I had were my business cards, no longer valid. I took one out, crossed out my old info, and wrote in my cell phone number. It was a little awkward having to explain why the card wasn't valid, like a credit card that had been declined. My business card had told the world (and me) who I was, why I was important, why you should know me. I'd been someone with a title: Geralyn Lucas, Lifetime Television, Director of Talent Relations and Corporate Communications. I'd had my own phone number (out of reach of my kids' and my husband's interruptions), an office with a door (and a lock, also kid- and husband-proof). Who was "I" now? That scared me. I had wanted to see if I could switch teams and spend time with my kids, not as an extracurricular activity, but as the main activity. But I still carried my card around, a vestige of who I used to be, and I could always write in my personal cell number if anyone asked for it. It offered me a sort of half-life identity. Like a dying cell battery, there was a tiny bit of juice left in it. The more people asked me for my card (and I kept crossing out my old title and info and writing in my cell) the stranger and more demoralized I felt. I hated crossing something out and feeling so unprofessional in my presentation now that I was no longer actually a professional. I especially hated how long I had struggled over getting a new title, when now it was obsolete. I thought about how hard people I knew worked to make partner or to get from VP level to senior VP level, as if "senior" totally changed them. They got more money and more responsibility, and all because of one word on a small card.

Who I used to be and who I was now seemed to blur, and my entire identity felt body-snatched. My business card had told me who I was, and without it I was measuring my worth based on how good my Floam project was that day. Whatever I had done in my career boiled down to the info on that little card, so small and rectangular, almost like a tiny headstone in a cemetery. It had defined my life, and by default it would be my obituary. This little card was all I had ever seemed to be. I started reading obits for ideas for my new business card. The first one I found: cat lover. I'm allergic. My former title had sustained me 24/7 and told me exactly who I was. There were e-mails and texts and calls to remind me. If I'd thought I was someone else for even a few hours, I was quickly sucked back into the magnetic field of that business card—the guiding, pulsing force in my life.

I finally figured out that I needed a new business card, but the problem was that without anyone telling me what my position was, I actually had no idea what to have printed on it. How did I want to sum up who I was, now that I was no longer a title in an organization? I could have declared my skills, like a "writer, producer" kind of card. I could have created a "calling card" with just my contact info. I was completely terrified about how to define myself in such a monumental way.

I'd had cancer and gone through horrible treatments; surviving that was a huge credential. But what else had I done? What was my worth? My *work* credentials felt so *yesterday*, now that I wasn't in my job. What was left when that job fell away and stopped? How should I present myself to the world? I decided that I wanted to be authentic in this stage of my life, and eliminate anyone who might try to befriend me because of where I worked or what I could do for him. Losing my job would be my reinvention moment. There was no looking back on my former titles. Telling people what I used to do felt very past tense and like I was trying to network, and I didn't want to give the impression that I was looking for work. I wanted to be present, in the moment, exactly where I was in my life, and I wanted to own exactly what I was doing.

I just wanted to be myself for once in my life. I didn't want to put on airs about all the great projects I was developing for the future. I wanted to focus on my kids, and so for a quick minute I thought the calling card solution would work—my name and contact info. There would be an air of mystery around it. I'd heard that celebrities had calling cards. It felt classy.

But then I was inspired to go deeper and be even more real. Aside from the Floam creations, my biggest accomplishment lately was being a mom. I loved spending time with my kids, except that sometimes being a mom got in the way of being a mom. There were so many forms to fill out for school, visits to pediatricians, camp trunks to pack, so many details of parenting. Right then, Hayden was mastering the potty, and the process had started to feel like a real boss/employee dynamic. "Ouch, you're wiping too hard," he'd complain after I tried to get that perfect wipe. It wasn't now about earning a promotion; it was the more existential concept of taking true pride in my work.

Freud said we need work to make us happy. The communist worker was supposed to feel a certain pride in the work he did, no matter how small, since it was contributing to a greater societal good. I was a tushy wiper, and I was going to be a damn good one. I was part of the circle of life, like in *The Lion King*. Gone were the days of bonus checks, glowing job evaluations, and thank-you lunches at fancy restaurants. Now I just had wiping.

After one very long day of mommydom, Hayden came over to me with his underwear still around his ankles after he'd flushed the potty with great flourish. He must have sensed my sadness and my lack of purpose these days. "Mommy, is wiping my tushy your favorite job ever?" I thought about all of the ass I kissed on my way up the corporate ladder: the mean ass, the skinny ass, the entitled ass, and then there was this chubby-cheeked angel.

It was very humbling, to be performing such sacred yet menial labor. It *was* my favorite job . . . but I had a flash of entering the gates of the White House and of hanging with Taylor Swift during a shoot. My new business card, if I got one printed: Tushy Wiper. But I wanted something more distinguishing to prove that I was earnest, that I took it seriously, and that I still had game.

Geralyn Lucas. Wiper *Extraordinaire*. The addition gave it a bit of panache. It was a wink and a nod that I did hard work and did it well. It also seemed low-key, yet upwardly mobile.

The moment to debut my new life and try out my new title appeared. I was at a very important TV party where I should have been networking with all my former colleagues. Everyone was gathered around the few famous people there. Geraldo Rivera looked at me as if he knew me, but couldn't place how. I had a fabulous conversation with a TV star. I was suggesting what her next pieces should be. She asked me for my card.

"I'm just a tushy wiper now. I don't carry a card," I sort of mumbled.

"There's someone you *must* meet," she said, and she was absolutely determined.

She introduced me to her husband, a stay-at-home dad.

In a party full of VIPs the two wipers were networking.

We compared notes about wiping, but then we started to talk about how nice it was to be out of the house and have a glass of wine after a whole day of being the garbage. It felt so real. We had a genuine spark; there was no ulterior motive for work advancement, no false promises about having lunch in the future. We just compared notes on how hard it was to be a parent, and how our spouses didn't get it. Sure, we missed our offices, but there was a je ne sais quoi about being there for someone, being vulnerable for another person. The endless meaningless tasks of the day added up to some gestalt I couldn't describe and neither could he. I was tired, I'd gained a muffin top, but I'd also gained some perspective about myself: I could exist without a business card. I had a new job, one that didn't pay, but made me feel so complete.

The next day Hayden seemed reluctant toward me when he headed for the potty. "Mommy, close the door. I need my privacy. I can do it now all by myself."

I was fired—no title, out of work again. I thought about how important my role had been. Hayden was now an independent little guy, and I had definitely had a hand in it. Maybe my greatest work to date.

I still experience PTSD because my job actually left me, went off to LA, like a boyfriend. I fantasized that my job would miss me so much, not be able to go on without me, beg me to come to LA. I pretended that my job couldn't live without me. But my job had met someone new.

One day, after a long session of Floam, Hayden and I were walking home. The feeling of having nowhere to be hit me. At first it was scary, that no one in the office needed me, that I wasn't being summoned to a meeting. But I looked down and saw Hayden's little hand holding my wrist, pulling me toward a bright red firehouse door.

"Should I knock, Hayden?"

"Yes! Mommy, I want to say hi to the firemen!"

Mommy wanted to say hi to some nice firemen too. It had been a bit isolating hanging with my son and all his friends.

I hoisted Hayden up and he rang the bell. It was a very loud ring, and I was worried that maybe we would be disturbing their important work. But a tall, redheaded, blue-eyed firefighter answered the door promptly. His name tag said MIKE and he seemed thrilled to have company.

"My son and I wanted to thank you for keeping our neighborhood so safe, right, Hayden?"

Hayden sprinted as fast as he could toward the awesomely huge, shiny red fire truck. Mike ran after Hayden, scooped him up in his arms, and climbed up behind the steering wheel. With Hayden on his lap, he demonstrated how to honk the horn. He even extended an arm for me to join them in the front seat of the fire truck. Mike was as hot as the fires he was called to, but he was also sweet. Watching Hayden awed by the station, Mike seemed to puff out his chest a bit more and feel even more important.

I got to honk the horn too, and it blasted straight to my brain. In my old life I was on a conveyor belt, moving too fast to step off. I was moving too fast to take time to stop into firehouses on a whim; I was always at a corporate job. Any free time, I was thinking about work.

It felt so good to have this little adventure, to meander and let life seep in, so slowly that I almost didn't notice. And my relationship with Meredith, who had been my boss and my friend, had morphed into a friendship that became even closer. What I'd thought was the biggest disappointment in my life—losing my job—turned into a window of opportunity for change. And there was even more change on the way.

CHAPTER 8
Mom/Daughter/Mother

I should have played more dress-up with her. I should have played more Barbies. I should have gone to more of her ballet classes. I should have pushed her more on the swings, because before I knew it Skye was twelve years old and leaving for her fourth summer at sleep-away camp. It didn't seem possible that my little girl who loved bubble baths was once again packing a toiletry kit and a trunk.

The large camp bus is parked on Fifth Avenue at Eighty-Fifth Street with its motor humming, as Skye boards and disappears inside. The deep smoky-gray glass windows are the total opposite of the clear glass box she was delivered to me in—these windows are impossible to see through, like my tween daughter.

I smell the exhaust from the idling engine and realize with a bit of anxiety that I can't see in to check on her, like I did before through the nursery glass. The first time Skye and I officially "separated" at nursery school was unbelievably painful. I hid behind a car and watched her leave the school with her class: Like all the other children, her little wrist was tucked through a loop of rope that was connected to a long rope that was connected to the teacher. She and the other kids were tethered to the teacher so they wouldn't stray off when they walked down the New York city block toward the park. She had entered the big world without me, and *she* was okay but *I* wasn't. I should have listened to those people who told me to enjoy Skye even more as the adorable baby and toddler she'd been.

I can't see through the glass of the camp bus window at all. It's the kind of glass made for paranoid people like celebrities who want to look out, but don't want to be seen. Or for kids who don't want to see their parents, when their parents are desperate for one last glance. It is a sort of privacy glass, a curtain between us. I know Skye can see me through the glass from her side, but I know she's not looking out. In fact, I know she's turned her head as far away from the window as possible, and she will keep her head turned to deliberately not see me and wave.

While Tyler uses his big muscles to lift her humongous trunk into the storage compartment of the bus, I decide to sneak onto the bus one last time. I want to give Skye one more hug. I walk up the steep stairs at the front of the bus and the cool air-conditioning hits my face. I hesitate a moment before taking the final step up and think of an excuse for being here: bug spray. I can't believe how panicked I am. I try to be brave. I am a breast cancer survivor. When I get past the bus driver, I realize suddenly that I've entered a strange world where all the kids have their headphones on, zoning off to music—except one. My daughter has noticed me and removed hers, with a look of terror: I have invaded a sacred space, like stepping from the audience onto the stage.

"Um, I wondered, did you remember your bug spray?" It is obvious I am lying. Her death stare is scarier than Darth Vader's and I am definitely *not* getting a final hug. I backtrack down the steep steps, ashamed, and return to my former position: staring into the dark window where I know she is sitting, turned away from me.

Silly me, I will wave until the bus is four blocks away and I can't even smell the fumes anymore. It hits me: As quickly as she came into my life, she'll be leaving it. Parenthood means still waving good-bye while your child is looking away, as far away as possible. I wish all the parents who told me to enjoy Skye when she was young had prepared me for *this* moment. Maybe then I would have hugged her even harder while she let me.

The trunk purchase; schlepping the trunk home; filling up the trunk with tube socks, flashlights, a soap holder, shorts, towels, sheets; ordering the SKYE LUCAS iron-on name labels that had to be applied to every item that could take the heat. Those labels never did stick when ironed, so they had to be sewed on: I made sure they stuck for her; I made sure that if she lost something, it would come back to her. And after all that labeling work, she won't look at me from the camp bus. I want to label her with my name and cell phone number and address to make sure she is always returned to me safely. I'm worried her label will fall off and she won't come back. I don't know how to stick it on so it stays. I am sending her out into the world, like a boomerang, hoping she will always come back to me after a brief interlude of separation.

Tyler and I are not allowed to hear her voice while she's at camp—no phone calls, just letters and e-mails and one visiting day after two weeks.

I think it's even harder for Tyler than it is for me, and I *hate* having to say good-bye again on visiting day. It is torture. I hug Skye so hard that I step on her exposed toes in her Birkenstock sandals.

"Mom, *ouch*! You stepped on my toe!"

When I look down and see her blue-painted toenails, for a moment I recall so vividly her tiny infant foot in a footsy pajama. I see her trying to stand up in her starter walking shoes from Stride Rite, the white orthopedic-looking ones that cover her ankles to give her support. I see her in first position in her scuffed ballet slippers with the laces that never stayed tied, and her chubby legs that seemed shoved so tightly into the pink tights that the tights might burst. I see her shiny Mary Janes that she refused to take off when she went to bed.

She pulls away and I remember the days after she learned to walk, tumbling toward me with her outstretched arms. There are so many shoes between us now. "Please, one more hug." I am begging her before we have to get into the car for the eight-hour ride back to Manhattan.

"Mom, stop!"

There is a strange barrier between us now. It is our . . . bras? Through the padding I try to feel her heartbeat. Mine is racing, like I can't believe she is mine. Like the first boy I kissed, I want to hold on to her to keep her forever. I try to push closer but again all that bra padding is in my way. I remember when I was convinced I couldn't have a baby, but then I heard her heartbeat at eleven weeks, in a hospital exam room, with a microphone pressed to my belly. I want to describe to her how I felt when I heard her heartbeat for the first time and how I need to feel her heartbeat now. How can I show her how much I love her without annoying her? I want our relationship to have no secrets, but Skye wants privacy. My miracle daughter has become *a little bit* mean.

It's when Skye is really nice to me these days that I get suspicious. "Hi, Mom. I mean Mommyyyyyy . . . ?" Her voice sounds like she wants a sweater. How do I describe Sweater Voice? Marilyn Monroe has nothing on my daughter. Picture Marilyn, all breathy and seductive singing, "Happy Birthday, Mr. President. . . ." Now imagine Skye as Marilyn asking me for a sweater. It is sort of a song. Flirty, breathy, staring straight into my eyes, she starts the seduction. "Mommy, I need a sweeeeaaattterrrrr. Mommmmy, everyone got another sweaaaater. Everyone!"

I want to cover my ears. Instead, I try reason: "How about the one we just bought?"

"It doesn't fit me anymore."

I fill in the blanks. Even though last week she couldn't live without it, this week she can't stand it. It's as if her very life hinges on buying the new sweater. I am tempted to tell her the story of the belt, and how no material object will compare with love, but then she starts in with her Leggings Voice. I know it is not her fault. She probably got the shopping gene from me. The Sweater Voice has such a siren wail; I can't turn away from it. My brain is in hand-to-hand combat to stop . . . THE SWEATER VOICE.

Where exactly is she wearing all these sweaters? Part of me is envious, because where are all these fabulous places she has to go? All these people she needs to look brand-new to? My sweaters are stretched and sagging and have some moth holes. But maybe that sweater will finally make her happy and solve all her problems. That sweater is seducing me too, like the belt. I will buy that sweater for her. And even though it is summer, I will buy that sweater because there is air-conditioning and I don't want her to catch a cold. If that sweater will complete her, then it will complete a tiny piece of me that yearns to be the yarn on her body. I want to be that close again, without my trying to hug her and having her push me away or duck.

She won't even let me see her naked. Her back is turned when she is changing, putting on the new sweater after she clasps the bra with the padding. I want to tell her, "But I made you! You made me vomit every morning, pee when I laughed, and made men not look at me. Please at least be nice. For like five minutes? Please don't look at me like you are mortified we are related. Like you can't believe we ever could be related, because I fed you via an umbilical cord and we share mitochondrial DNA, the smallest chromosome of you, the first significant part of your human genome to be sequenced, inherited solely from me. You owe me . . . *your life.*"

. . . .

*A*nd then one day comes a milestone I never thought I could reach: I have lived long enough to witness my daughter become a young woman.

"Mom, I'm sorry, but I just got my period. That's why I'm so cranky." Skye is blaming her moodiness on her hormones. My baby girl can be a mom herself, and the older she gets, the more she'll need me—to protect her from boys, from her friends, from everything else that might happen in her life. I know she thinks that I am the problem, but I need to convince her that it is my job to find the solutions.

"Sweetie, why are you so mean to me?" I'm looking at her blue eyes, which match the sky, and I just keep staring in disbelief that I had something to do with this beauty. My eyes are filling with tears but I'm willing myself not to cry because that will make her feel guilty. All I can say is, "Mommy loves you so much."

And all she can say back is, "I know, it's just really hard having hormones!" She is pleading with me to understand her lapses into meanness.

"Trust me, it's worse *not* having them."

"What does that mean?" She does seem genuinely confused.

"Mommy has had hormones, and now they are leaving. You are menstruating. I am menopausing."

How could so much hormonal chaos occur under one small Manhattan apartment roof? It's a very sick but sort of funny trick that just as girls become meanest, their moms get craziest. What exactly did God have in mind with this hormonal collision course?

But that is wrong, and I know I have "enmeshment" issues with my daughter. I blur where I end and she begins. I'm too dependent on her approval and her love. I need to respect her; she is her own young lady trying to be independent, and I need to respect boundaries. But then I want to shout, "Twenty hours of contractions with no medicine, and screaming women all around me, just to bring you here—and guess who held my hand when I cried?"

My mother.

I'm sure I was never mean to my mom. Where could my daughter have learned this horrible behavior?

"Trust me, you were worse to me." My mom is very direct when I ask her about how I was as a teen. I have no memory of my own horrible behavior, but I do trust her because until she told me about how I had been to her, this is how I answered the phone when she called: "Hi. What? I'm busy."

Then my daughter did that to me, even though Skye is always nice when her friends call. The way I feel now about Skye is probably how my mother used to feel about me.

Skye has just closed her bedroom door on me. I was in the room when she was born, and now all she does is close the door for privacy.

"Mom, please, I just need some privacy."

"Privacy?" I want to ask her through the closed door. "You lived inside of me!" I wish I could open the door she just slammed and tell her about when I first held her. Tell her about how I used to read her *Pat the Bunny* at least five times in a row, sitting in the comfy overstuffed chair in the corner. And each time she touched the bunny, I clapped.

I am staring at her closed door when I hear my cell phone ring. MOM flashes across the screen.

"What? I'm really busy. . . ."

"Hi, sweetie, how are you? I wanted to hear how that meeting went for you today."

"Mom, how did you deal with me? I need some help with Skye."

"She'll come back to you."

Why has it taken thirty years for me to learn to be nice to my mom? I don't know if I'll live long enough for Skye to learn to be nice to me.

I do remember one horrible time I was being mean to my mom, and I wasn't a teen. She had taken a train in from Philadelphia to be with me at my first chemo treatment. I was a wreck because my doctor was away at a conference, and some doctor I didn't know had to give it to me. I had spent the entire night *before* the chemo vomiting in anticipation. The doctor came into the room and explained the process, and then she asked my mom to step out for a minute.

"Do you know how awful you're being to your poor mother? Your mom is suffering too. Imagine how hard it is for her to see you going through this. This is a tragedy for her too. Stop being mean to your mother! She's here for you."

The doctor yelled at *me* before my chemo!

I think I was probably taking out all my anxiety on my mother before my treatment. She was my pincushion before I got the needles, and it wasn't fair to her. I was a grown woman and I was being mean to my mom. How could I expect my daughter to be nice to me if I was so mean to my own mom? Is it just in our DNA, an inescapable, programmed Darwinian behavior between mothers and daughters? Is there a cure?

My mom is calling.

"Mommy, hi!" I am trying to sound as delighted as I really am to hear her voice. I know how dependent I am on my own daughter's moods and how happy I feel when Skye is happy.

But why does Skye jiggle the bottom of my arms and tell me I have back fat and give me the Darth Vader death stare when I dance? Lately she has nothing but my faults to talk to me about. Otherwise, she is a tween of few words. A typical conversation:

Me: Sweetie, what did you have for lunch today?

Skye: Food.

Me: What are you wearing to the birthday party tonight?

Skye: Clothes.

Me: Who did you hang out with at school today?

Skye: People.

Suddenly, she opens her mouth as if to share something, and I want to cover my ears so I don't hear the sweater song. It starts with "Mommy."

"Mommy . . ." I am prepared to say no to the sweater. "Cuddle me!"

I haven't heard that in so long.

She is my baby again, lying on my bed with me, nestled in my arms, but her toes are way farther down—she's almost taller than I am. I pull her closer, like I've finally caught this little butterfly that has grown her wings and is flying away.

I can't believe she is mine: I smell her highlighted hair; I want to brush it and put on her favorite headband with the flower, which she used to wear every day. I can't choose her accessories anymore. She used to be my little accessory, tucked into a BabyBjörn like a handbag I slung over me. I could put bows in her hair and people would admire how cute she was. She would smile at everyone, even at me.

She tells me in between cuddles, "I'm sorry that I'm mean to you. You are just so annoying sometimes."

And I *am* annoying, but not as annoying as I remembered *my* mom. Skye has every right to be embarrassed at the way I dance. I've become an embarrassing dresser too. I make mistakes as a mom. I even forgot Special Tutu Day at her ballet class when she was little—I hope she doesn't remember that now. All the little girls around us were wearing amazing special tutus. I had just run from work and totally forgotten that Skye was allowed to wear a special tutu over her pink leotard and tights that day.

"Mom, why can't you remember things like other moms do?"

Another mom in the locker room saw the confrontation and offered me her daughter's special tutu for Skye to wear to her class. In that instant in the ballet locker room I forgave my mom for everything wrong she ever did. Ever. The next week I sent Skye to stand at the school bus stop when it was an "in service" day and there was no school. I pray my daughter will forgive me for all my mistakes and for being so annoying.

I remembered her, only eighteen months old, wearing a white lace dress with a pink velvet bow in her hair, chomping on a Chinese sparerib with her two front teeth. She was giggling so hard that people in the restaurant would stop eating, look up, and start to laugh too. She began pounding her sparerib on the table, laughing even more. One couple came over to our table—I thought maybe they were going to complain about the noise, but instead they asked to squeeze her rosy cheeks.

"Enjoy her. You won't believe how fast she'll grow up. Ours just left for college."

Another day out in New York, I was pushing her in her stroller down the frozen-food aisle at Gristedes supermarket and an older lady was shuffling by with a walker. She stopped me when she saw then-two-year-old Skye, bundled up in a bright yellow floral raincoat with a matching hat.

"I'd give anything to trade my walker for your carriage," she said wistfully. "I miss my little girl."

I miss my little girl too. For a moment I see Skye wearing the pink "Mommy" nightgown that was mine, the one that matched her own child-size pink nightgown. Her legs were so tiny then, but they're longer than mine now. I'm getting to watch my little girl grow up.

I know I have to let her grow up. I have to believe that she will come back, even though she isn't labeled. She's not mine anymore; she's hers—and that's okay, I guess. I so badly want to knock down my daughter's door when she closes it, but I know that for now she needs her room to grow.

I really try to fit my arms all the way around her for the cuddle, and one arm brushes her bra padding as I push her long, highlighted hair aside so I can press my cheek against hers before she has time to pull away. I have seen her permanent teeth grow in, but she has so much more growing up to do, and my prayers for her have evolved: Please let her grow boobs as big as she wants; please let her breasts be safe, and never, ever make her have to lose one. Please don't let her worry that my fate is hers. Please make her just a little nicer to me *sometimes*. Please make her think I'm a good mom. Please, Victoria's Secret, make thinner padding in your bras so I can feel the hug more. And please let Skye's daughter be as mean to her as she was to me as I was to my mom. *Please* let me live to see that.

CHAPTER 9
Red Velvet Cupcake

*M*y usually modest thirteen-year-old daughter has let me come into the dressing room with her at Victoria's Secret, where she is shopping for bras. It is as if we have crossed a threshold, being inside the dressing room, finally on the same side. She used to scream at me through the door, and hand stuff underneath. She used to hide her breasts from me. I start having a rush of PTSD because I see the word *PINK* in bright pink sequins everywhere, and my annual mammogram is tomorrow. Victoria's Secret pink is definitely not breast-cancer pink, and that's how I want to keep it for Skye: sexy, lacy, and push-up. This feels like such a normal mother-daughter moment we are sharing, until I anticipate the mammogram, and I get a bit nauseated in the all-pink dressing room surrounded by so many bras.

"Mom, can I get this one too? I love it. . . . Does it look okay?" I focus on Skye, and the white lace bra she's trying on hints of the bandage I had on my chest after my mastectomy.

In the mirror she is so perfect and innocent. I feel my eyes watering and I don't want her to see the tears.

"Mom, did you hear me? Are you okay?"

"I'm fine, I just remembered that I have my mammogram tomorrow."

I'm trying to sound as routine as the mammogram is supposed to be.

Skye is still admiring the push-up bra, lost in her image of herself. I'm surprised when she asks, "Do you want me to come with you?" She is still looking in the mirror, scrunching her nose a bit at her reflection, and I wonder if she understands the implications of her offer.

"I'd really like that," I say. And I would.

I'm still terrified that my boobs will kill me. And now I'm terrified about my daughter's growing breasts. That was my biggest fear when I had her: Would she have my eyes, my bad math skills, and my breast cancer? I could almost faint picturing Skye someday being told she has breast cancer. The possibility of Skye with an IV in her arm from chemo, a bandage on her breast, is making me so queasy I sit down on a pile of bras to catch my breath.

Skye has picked out ten bras for herself, which I whittle down to six. She is both beautiful and awkward in her new bras, so on the cusp of womanhood. I can't decide whether she is still my little girl or a grown woman, this poised young lady, her blue eyes sparkling now with more intelligence than mischief.

Later that day, when I tell my friend Betsy that Skye has offered to come with me to my mammogram and that I've said yes, she thinks I've crossed a line I shouldn't have. "What if something bad happens? She can't handle that. Why did you do that to her?"

I feel guilty, but something inside me knows that Skye is ready. Maybe she's picturing herself in that mammogram room someday, and when she's in that room, I want her to remember my courage.

I am trying to find that courage in the cab ride over to the radiologist. My palms are sweating. Skye is holding my hand, and I hope she doesn't feel the sweat. You cannot wear deodorant to a mammogram, and I'm worried I smell. Armpit odor definitely wouldn't match my game face. I need to be a role model for my daughter, but I want to smell good too.

When I'm handed the clipboard to fill in my medical history, I hesitate a bit when I write "mastectomy, 27 years old" to answer the question, "Have you had breast surgery?" I look around the waiting area, where my daughter is seated, and I see anxiety on all the faces, and it just smells like bad news. I wonder why each woman is here. Is it a suspicious lump, family history screening, or routine mammogram? Skye seems so out of place, so young and tender and her face so carefree. I wish Skye never had to be in this waiting room, but she'll need to have mammograms, especially with my history.

Getting a mammogram is like waiting for a ride at Disneyland: You get past the front waiting room only to find more waiting before the main event. I am led to the back area where each patient has her own private little cubby that the staff calls a locker room, with a full-length mirror, a chair, and some paper towels to wipe off any goop left from a sonogram, if needed. There are magazines on a side rack and even a place to hang your coat. Today I'm assigned to locker room 3 and given a key to let me in and out. Skye is allowed to come in with me. The walls are a muted pink, but with a much different vibe than the Victoria's Secret dressing room, where it feels like a boob fiesta. This small locker room is more like a breast library—very hushed and serious. This pink is a subtle and dignified pink, not a happy push-up bra pink. I take off everything above the waist.

Skye is staring at my reconstructed breast and the scar from the mastectomy.

"Mom, does your scar ever hurt?"

"It used to but not anymore."

My daughter looks at me a beat too long and I realize I am being examined. "I feel bad for you that everyone can see your scar."

I quickly put on one of the pink cotton robes.

Skye is embarrassed about my scar when it peeks out from bathing suits and dresses. I want to tell her that it has become a part of me now; my scar is a secret mother-daughter lesson that I have never quite known when to share.

But then someone with a clipboard calls out, "Mrs. Lucas."

"Good luck, Mom," Skye says as she heads out of our locker cubby back toward the waiting area, and the clipboard person leads me back to the mammogram room. I am cold and shivering as I untie my gown and step up to the machine's chilly plates. The mammography technician tells me her name is Sandra. I watch Sandra take in the long faded-red mastectomy scar running down the right side of me, just the way Skye looked at it.

Sandra pushes me closer to the mammogram machine and turns me so my "real" left breast is resting on the bottom plate.

"Pretend you're not here," she encourages me, sensing my nerves, as she is manipulating, squeezing, repositioning, and squeezing again. She is clearly a pro, but I wonder how she can stay in this room every day, this room of possible bad news and a big scary machine that holds the future.

"Don't breathe. Just hold the position. Close your eyes."

My breast is being squeezed hard and pancake flat. You never realize just how flat your breast can become until it's in the machine. Sandra escorts me back into my little locker room, and the harsh fluorescent lighting is so not flattering when I look in the mirror.

All the years I've looked into these locker room mirrors during my annual mammograms, just praying to grow old enough to have wrinkles—and now I'm sad to see my prayers answered. This morning I applied thick foundation to erase the sunspots and broken capillaries on my face and to smooth out the pores that seem to be growing larger by the second. My face is falling and looks like it needs a lot of sleep or more foundation. Lately, my makeup routine has become a cover-up routine, and I take it seriously. I know now what an older woman means when she says she has to "put on her face."

As I keep staring into the mirror, it's clear that, sadly, I've lost the wonder of my cancer gratitude moment. After cancer I thought that the thrill of returning to life and being well would stick, and that I would always be satisfied with being healthy and growing old. Not true.

I am now—at forty-five—dissatisfied. And today I feel even worse about it. I feel guilty knowing that I should *only* feel lucky that I have my health and my hair and the wrinkles I prayed for. I feel shallow because I'm disappointed that I'm aging, and sagging.

It would be good for Skye to see that a woman can age gracefully, especially her own mother, so why can't I embrace my wrinkles like a badge of honor, a badge that in my case especially would say "I survived"?

I make another promise to myself: If there's no cancer, I will appreciate my wrinkles. I will be thankful that I'm okay and smile when I look in the mirror. I will not complain about my pores. I will love everything, in all its healthy glory.

A clock ticks in my head while I'm waiting for the radiologist to read the images. Since my daughter is with me at this screening, the question is even scarier: *Will I go back to my life, or back to the operating room?*

Skye's breasts are out of context in this place. They are part of a fun new chapter in her life, a chapter of growth and possibility and excitement. I remember being thirteen years old, and so badly wanting to wake up with boobs. I'm sure if Skye could water hers and sprinkle them with breast food, she would. But there's no magic formula to growing breasts. It is all just so mysterious.

I look at myself in the mirror, open my gown, and stare at mine. I miss them—the way they used to be before cancer. Almost every woman I know wants her breasts either smaller or bigger, a reduction or implants. I have only met one woman *ever* who loved hers exactly the way they were. I want to tell my friends, "Your boobs are healthy! Enjoy!" I want to tell every woman who hates her breasts to love them, because they might disappear. I always wanted bigger breasts; now they are bigger from my reconstruction, but suddenly the breast I had to give up is something I long for. All these years later, I still dream about the smaller breast I lost. It was mine. It was perfect. I never loved it then, but I miss it so much now.

There is a knock at my locker cubby door. Skye has come to check on me, and we squeeze in together, facing the mirror.

"You okay?" She looks worried.

"Yeah, we just have to wait a little while to see if they're normal."

"Phew!" Skye says, squeezing some invisible pimple on her face. There are times Skye appears confident, but she's also terrified of zits and she hates her freckles. She is pure thirteen-year-old swagger mixed with meltdowns.

"Mom, I'm thinking about getting a blue streak in my hair. In the back, so it's not obvious."

"I don't think that'll go over so well with your school and Ms. Hoffman."

"Mo-om," she says. "Everyone has one."

Hair is a big deal to Skye. She's always stocking our bathroom shelves with new hair products that promise more volume, shine, and more *hair*.

"Can I get blond highlights?"

After the blue hairstreak request, blond highlights seem so reasonable that at first I'm sort of relieved. But my daughter doesn't have light hair. She's deep brunette.

"Honey, your hair is beautiful. Don't dye it until the day comes when you have to cover the gray. I wanted to be blond all my life, but now that I'm gray I dye my hair the exact shade I always was: black."

How much money am I now paying once a month to have my hair dyed to the exact same color it *always* was despite my never having loved my natural color? I was embarrassed that my hair was so dark and black and different—and all the girls used to call me "witch" and chase me around the playground and pull my hair *hard*. I lament all that time I wasted hating my hair. After chemo, all I wanted was the exact hair that I had never appreciated. My wig had to look exactly like the hair I'd had. I did *not* want the blond wig. But then I don't want to scare Skye by making her think about when I had cancer, before she was born.

The clock is ticking. What is taking Sandra so long? Was my mammogram normal? It is so hard waiting for my mammogram results, and my mind jumps around to everything that could be wrong on the film.

"Mrs. Lucas, we need some more images."

I hug Skye and I am led back to the mammogram machine, and when I put my breast between the plates again, I try to think about other things I want to tell my daughter before it might be too late. Like: Skye, stop trying so hard to grow up, because when you're older, you might miss being young. When Skye and I shop together, Skye flees the juniors' department because she thinks it's cheesy and not mature enough. She is shopping in the women's department, and I have to admit I sneak into juniors' and drool because the clothes feel really hot, and I want to see what the tweens and teens are wearing, to inspire my wardrobe so I feel current. I'm not alone. Most of Skye's friends' moms wear tight jeans that are *so not* mom jeans, and they seem to be trying to look like their tween daughters.

I am tempted to make an announcement at the clothing store. I would like to get onto the PA system and yell, "Ladies, girls: Stay in your own department! Ladies, please return to women's. . . . Girls, please return to juniors'. Right *now*!"

Sandra escorts me back to my locker room, where Skye is making a face at the mirror.

"Hey, Mom." Skye hugs me so tight it makes me want to get mammograms more often.

"Skye, you look especially beautiful today."

"Mom, please stop staring at me."

"I can't, you're so beautiful."

"I'm not, and don't stare. I am not beautiful. You just think that because you're my mom."

Somehow the fluorescent light makes me look yellow but my daughter look even more amazing. And for a moment it feels like an out-of-body experience watching my daughter and me in the mirror: I can't believe what I see.

Then Skye yells at the mirror, "I hate my freckles, Mom!" As if screaming at her freckles in the mirror might actually scare them away. "They are *so* annoying." My heart sinks: I think her freckles are gorgeous, like a painting on her skin. I want to remind Skye that her hero, Amelia Earhart, had freckles—but there's a problem. The history books report Amelia also *hated* her freckles and was incredibly self-conscious about them. My daughter learned about Amelia in school. When I was growing up, I worshiped Amelia Earhart too, and I wanted to break boundaries the way she had. The woman who broke barriers . . . hated her freckles? Even the glamorous, accomplished, and historic Amelia Earhart wanted desperately to change something about herself. No amount of glory could erase that longing.

This is what I'd like to say to Amelia: "Millions of women admire you, so *love* your freckles. They are cute and sexy and adorable. They make you seem real, as if you'd spent time in the sun. You loved to climb to the clouds and maybe you thought you could touch the sun. Flying so close to the sun causes freckles. They are yours. Own them, Amelia!"

Skye got her freckles from my mom. I recently found a photo of my mom when she was Skye's age, and she was so pretty I couldn't believe I was related to her. All that time when I was a teenager and I was embarrassed by her and mean to her—was this the same woman I tormented?

The snapshot was a black-and-white and she looked like an old-time movie star. I was sort of shocked by the glamour of the photo and of this woman I had known all my life and never really seen. I was excited to show the picture to her and Skye, and I expected Mom to blush and say something like "I drove the boys crazy." But when I did show it to her, she just stared and stared and seemed so sad. Finally she said, "I never felt pretty growing up."

"Whaaaat?" I almost shouted at her. How could she not have seen her own beauty? My mom got very quiet and looked like she was about to cry. She seemed shamed about what she was sharing with me, as if she were telling me a secret that hurt her very much.

"I was too skinny," Mom whispered, and she meant what she said.

"Too skinny? Who ever felt too skinny?" I was about to burst out laughing, because I was trying to diet, and wore Spanx; how could she say she'd been too skinny? Was it a joke? I couldn't believe being thin had made her feel ugly.

"When I grew up, people were supposed to be plump—*that's* what was beautiful. My mother always told me to drink milkshakes every day, but I stayed skinny. Today my skinny body would be considered a knockout." She looked away from the photo. "I hated those milkshakes, Skye."

Skye said, "Why did you hate them? I would *love* drinking vanilla milkshakes all the time."

"No, you wouldn't," Mom said. "They forced me to do it and it didn't help at all. But I feel beautiful right now. I'm almost seventy and it does take some work, you know; I get my nails done and my hair done once a week. But it's not really the appointments. I feel pretty now, more poised. I look at pictures from when I was young, like this one, and I see that I was so stiff. Now I'm relaxed and just myself."

She smiled at me and added, "But I still can't believe I made *you*." She was proud of Skye and me. It was making her feel good about herself. I couldn't tell her that I wasn't impressed with myself, because that might have robbed her of her pride. I couldn't tell her that I was embarrassed by what she'd said because I have yet to learn to relax and love myself.

"Mom, I can't believe I'm related to *you*. You are so cool." I never would have thought that one day I would think my mom was cool. Would Skye ever think that I was *cool* and not annoying?

My mother has a feather woven into her hair now, and she seems to walk differently. She's confident and has a swagger, a lot like Skye's, which makes her seem as if she's finally a very mature thirteen-year-old girl, with attitude and bright red nails. I look at my daughter and I wonder: Does any woman truly love to look in the mirror? Why don't women want to look like themselves? And why are women always pointing to other women they'd rather look like? Chances are that the *other women* that the first set of women are trying to look like are women who have done something to themselves to look like *someone else*. And so on and so on and so on.

Another knock at the locker door, and I pull my pink gown tighter.

"Mrs. Lucas, give me five more minutes." It is Sandra, and I am worrying.

Here's *the* secret I need to tell Skye after this mammogram:

The one time in my life when I felt most comfortable with my looks was during my cancer treatments, when all those ugly things happened to my outside.

I had to work hard to find things that weren't on the surface and weren't right there staring back at me from a mirror: my kindness, my brain, my family's love, my friends.

When I lost my pretty—was divested of it, like a turtle without its hard shell for protection—I was unrecognizable to myself and to people who knew me, but I was still somehow *me*. I felt like a cupcake without icing, but I was still a cupcake. A red velvet one—I didn't need the icing. It was a sort of existential moment, because then I discovered how to find something inside that could still be beautiful, that no scalpel could take away. I called it "inner cleavage," and it was my "game," and I had game even when my chest was stitched and oozing.

When there was nothing left on the outside, it was all inside of me, and I was shining because I knew that people had to really notice *me*. It was autumn when I had my chemo, and as the trees were losing their leaves, I was losing my trimmings, but I was still a tree.

I thought I had finally made peace with the mirror when I posed for a topless photo for a women's magazine, after my mastectomy. Skye would cringe—there was my scar for everyone to see. When the photographer showed me the image, it astounded me. Instead of focusing on my long diagonal scar, I saw my eyes and my courage. It was the first time I ever felt beautiful. That picture made me aware of my journey, and I really "saw" myself for the first time.

I thought the wonder of that moment would stay with me, and I would always see myself a bit differently. I was proud of the way I looked that autumn because it meant I was still there despite what I had lost. Yet all I wanted was to look exactly the way I had looked before cancer. I wanted to look like *me* again. The me I never appreciated.

"Okay, Mrs. Lucas," Sandra finally calls through the door. "You can get dressed and go back out to the waiting area."

I wonder if this is the moment my doctor will appear to tell me my cancer is indeed back. She finally comes into the locker area and knocks on the door while I am changing. I grab the pink gown I've just removed, hold it in front of my breasts for some modesty, and open the door.

"Your results are fine."

Skye hugs and kisses me. When we are waiting for the elevator, my daughter looks me up and down. "Mom, I really like your outfit today."

I decide I will wear this outfit every day because she likes it.

As we leave the building, I feel so elated, and not just because I had good results today. I feel great because Skye usually disapproves of my jeans, my armpit acne (is there really such a thing?), my muffin top. She seems bothered by *me*. She doesn't like the way I breathe (seriously) or the way I talk (too much). But today I thought she could finally see *me*, what I saw when my leaves fell off, when my outside fell away. Today I thought she could see inside of me, and nothing on my outside was bothering her now. I was healthy and okay.

That night I promise myself that every time I look in the mirror I'll see myself through my mom's adoring eyes (the "I can't believe I made you" lens of wonder) and through Skye's admiring gaze (the "Mom, I like your outfit" look of approval). I am my mom's daughter and my daughter's mom, and I will treasure those beautiful bookends and be aware that I'm the connection between those two beauties.

When Skye is a bit older, I will tell her about my autumn, when I lost my leaves. I will show her the picture of myself with the huge scar. I will teach her how to really love herself. For now, Skye approves of me, even though I don't fully approve of myself. I have always been afraid that my daughter would get my self-hate, my legs, my ass, and my breasts.

Please, Skye, don't get my cancer. Please love yourself, Skye, even though your mother wants . . . Botox.

. . . .

Before my mammogram, I had scheduled a Botox appointment, and even after my "love myself" therapy session with myself in the mirror of the pink locker room, I decide to keep it.

When I arrive at the plastic surgeon's office, he describes how I can look like "myself" again. It doesn't only involve the usual Botox, and he assumes I liked the way I looked to start with.

"Your cheeks, that fullness you used to have—we want to regain that."

I stare hard into the gorgeous antique hand mirror thinking, *I never realized that my cheeks had fullness, or that they were something I should have loved.* I'm willing to consider pain to make them what the doctor says they once were.

The doctor explains that he has come up with a treatment he calls "Wow" cheeks, which involve a filler type of injection. He is patenting it, publishing about it. Because when women look in the mirror for the first time after this treatment, they say, "Wow." Actually, they say, "WOW!" All caps, exclamation point.

I want to cry when the doctor tells me what these women say next: "*Yes!* That is *me*! This is exactly how I used to look. These are my cheeks again!" Sometimes, according to the doctor, they are so excited about looking like themselves again that they become very emotional and even cry. But I'll bet that secretly they were never, ever in love with their cheeks when they were thirteen. And even if they did love their cheeks, and in the unlikely event that before they lost them they said "WOW!" every time they looked in the mirror, I'll bet they hated their butts or their noses.

In the plastic surgeon's office I start to think about the word "WOW!" with an exclamation point, and it's bothering me. Because women, or at least the women I know, so rarely say it when they look in the mirror.

Imagine, for a moment, if on cue every woman in America screamed "WOW!" when she looked in the mirror. Like she was the best thing she'd ever seen in her entire life. "WOW!" would echo through bedrooms and mirrored department-store dressing rooms, and the sound would be so loud and exciting that it would ricochet off the crown of the Statue of Liberty, bounce along the New York City sidewalks, and even echo through New Jersey, Pennsylvania, Ohio, Indiana, Illinois, Iowa, Nebraska, and Denver, Colorado, on the way to the Grand Canyon. "WOW!" "WOW!" "WOW!"

I decide to pass on the "WOW!" cheeks and only get the Botox shots today. I want to work on my wow without the "WOW!" cheek procedure. The doctor pushes the Botox needle in, and I close my eyes and think about truly loving myself. A "WOW!" kind of love. *Of course* I am striving for the intellectual self-love, but I just want to look a bit better.

I remember seeing that love on my niece Stella's face at her ninth birthday party at a roller skating rink. Stella was skating solo to Katy Perry's "Firework." She was wearing the most amazing blue-and-green-striped dress and a disco-ball necklace, gliding around the rink with her curly blond hair flying. She even dipped down and extended one leg, doing a cool trick. I want her always to have that joy, always feel so happy to be herself.

When I was nine I felt the same way. What happened to make me lose my confidence? Where do our nine-year-old selves go? How do we destroy our spirits and how do we ever build them back? Can the Botox make mine reappear? The doctor hands me the mirror and I do look sort of amazing after that shot. The Botox really helps lift my face up and seems like a subtle, teeny bit of air freshener for my face.

I'm hesitant to let Skye know that I've gotten Botox shots but I tell her anyway.

"No problem, Mom. Whatever makes you happy."

She stares at my face intently to see if she can notice the difference. And then she realizes she has an angle. "Oh, does that mean I can get my ear cartilage pierced?"

The problem with being a mom is that I need to be my daughter's role model, but I still haven't learned what my own mom tried to teach me: Just love yourself. So I want to say this to Skye as my final lesson about beauty:

I am forty-three, and trying hard to fall in love with myself. You are thirteen, and have your whole life stretched out ahead of you. Maybe some of the confidence that my mom missed growing up, and that I'm still trying to find, will be there in our next generation of women—in you, Skye. And maybe my mom's journey toward her *newfound* confidence will inspire both of us.

When Skye looks in the mirror and finds that something is not right, which seems to be all the time now, I feel a pain sharper than the Botox needle. I want to help my daughter get past her self-criticism, but if I can't get past *mine*, how can I expect *her* to pull that off?

Here's my promise to you, Skye: I promise that I won't feel dread when I look in the mirror, only pure infatuation. I want to love me always and not lose any more time with myself. Years from now I don't want to look at a photo and say, "Wow! I never knew how amazing I really looked!" I want to say "WOW!" now.

Seventy-five percent of women hate looking in the mirror, and 39 percent report that it negatively impacts their self-confidence. I refuse to be one of those stats anymore. If I need a shot to get me there, at least I will get there. I promise I will get there, Skye. I am still the tree.

The red velvet cupcake without the icing.

The naked turtle.

Just a little bit tighter around the eyes and forehead.

CHAPTER 10
Romance Smackdown

*I*t is Valentine's Day, and there is a romance smackdown about to happen in my apartment between the two men in my life: my kindergarten son and my middle-aged husband. They are both pulling out all the stops to impress me. Skye, with her new interest in boys, doesn't care about any of the romance going on at home. She'd always been a daddy's girl, but now she's grown out of it, and this—in addition to his new competition—is making Tyler a bit edgy.

Hayden has been working on his handmade valentine at school for almost a week. Tyler, worried about Hayden's constant progress reports on the impending surprise, has told me that he has actually made a dinner reservation for the two of us. Wow, that hasn't happened in ages.

The love competition has been brewing for a while. Tyler seems almost jealous of Hayden's endless affection for me, and I think it's inspiring him to outdo himself this year.

To be honest, Hayden's dizzy mom-love takes the sting out of the waning romance between my husband and me. If I ever question my commitment to my husband, I know that there's another guy just waiting patiently, in my own apartment, playing *Star Wars* video games. Hayden has made his intentions very clear: "Mommy, I want Daddy to take me to a Really Big Mommy Store . . . to buy you a diamond wing so I can mawy you." Hayden is still working on his *R*'s with his speech therapist.

Tyler, seeking to trump Hayden in Valentine romance, buys me a beautiful pair of pearl earrings and takes me out for a lobster dinner—leaving Hayden at home with a babysitter. But that didn't compare to Hayden's present, a crooked red construction-paper heart with over-size, scrawled capital letters earnestly proclaiming his absolute devotion: "TO GERALYN LOVE HAYDEN." As he offered me this handmade heart with all its imperfections, my heart was officially his. Maybe it was seeing that he'd handprinted my name that made me swoon. I thought about every love letter I'd ever received, how the boys had written my name, and how I'd analyzed their handwriting for clues to their personalities. Hayden's bold letters spelled it out for me. His handwriting style revealed no agendas, no games, and no secrets. Just bold block letters he'd worked so hard to write. This guy wore his heart on his sleeve; he was actually giving it to me. Forget the bad boys I had chased, and the ones who'd played hard to get. Hayden is my new ideal, and as a bonus, I know exactly what this guy's mommy issues are.

I think that deep down Tyler is happy that his son is so in love with me. After all, he was in love with *his* mom, and I took that to heart when I married him. Everyone knows that a man treats his wife like his mom. That seems harmonious and healthy. But lately Tyler has noticed how much better Hayden treats me than *he* does, and how Hayden courts me. And I have noticed how differently Tyler treats me *now* than he did in our courtship phase.

The comparisons are jarring:

Hayden runs to greet me with a kiss every time I walk in the door.

Tyler barely calls out a weak "hey" from his position on the sofa, without moving, to greet me.

Hayden insists on walking me out to the elevator every time I leave the apartment and gives me a kiss and a long hug. He releases me, staring straight into my eyes and begs, "Mommy, when will you be home?" Hayden holds the elevator door for me and says, "Ladies forst." He is still having a hard time pronouncing his vowels properly.

Tyler lets the door hit me.

Hayden is more adorable and our love is new and exciting. I am much more "in love" with Hayden. The "in love" thing is a dangerous condition; some have likened being in love to a brain's being on opiates. Tyler and I have been together nearly eighteen years, so there is a certain love fatigue that's setting in, so different from the "in love" phase.

In couple's therapy, I tell my therapist that my romance with Hayden has ruined my husband for me. That Hayden has made me believe in romantic love again. He notices everything good about me, unlike my husband, who only seems to notice what is wrong.

Hayden tells me, "Mommy, you look so stywish," and he'll always check me over approvingly before I'm headed out.

Tyler will say, "Did you brush your hair? Why are you wearing *that*?" My husband will always find a flaw on the way out to a party.

Hayden will snuggle up against me at night, with his Bun-Bun stuffed rabbit and blanket between us, content just to cuddle with a sweet smile on his face. I turn my back on Tyler to cuddle with Hayden, and Tyler says, "How come you never cuddle me anymore?" Tyler can't just cuddle without wanting something more. And he gets grumpy: There are Legos all over the place, the dishwasher hasn't been unloaded, and I didn't bring the mail up. Such a huge turn-on!

Hayden will save some of his snack for me and bring it home after school.

Tyler will eat the last bite.

Hayden doesn't want anything from me except an occasional Oreo and a *Star Wars* Lego set. He doesn't want to change me, and thinks that I am perfect. He needs me in ways that make me feel powerful, not vulnerable. And no Austrian-crystal belt or even my diamond engagement ring could ever compare to the sight of Hayden, hunched in his little school cubby, waiting for me to pick him up.

The love I have for Hayden and the change in my relationship with my husband has me so confused about love. I miss the wooing stage with my husband. But I know that I've changed *too*.

When Hayden coughs, it sounds adorable and I play Florence Nightingale. "Poor baby," I coo. I let Hayden cough on my face all night, and I gently wipe the phlegm off his face and mine.

When Tyler coughs, I demand he cover his mouth; I duck as if he is contagious, like I want to wear an H1N1 mask for viral protection.

When Hayden farts, I think it's adorable. When Tyler has skid marks in his underwear, it bothers me so much that I hate to think of my laundry even having to mingle with his in the same hamper.

When Hayden takes one bite of a pickle and puts the pickle back in the jar, I have no problem and might even finish it myself. When Tyler does that, I consider it contamination.

When Hayden aims for the potty, he often misses and leaves a trail. It is so cute to think of his tiny stream of glittering pee-pee arching up like a rainbow and just missing the bowl. When Tyler misses the bowl, I request him to Clorox.

When Hayden leaves the toilet seat up, I always put it down for him and don't say anything. It's so heavy that I worry he might crush his little fingers if he tries to put it down himself. When Tyler leaves the toilet seat up, I make a point of calling him in to the bathroom to reprimand him.

I am caught between two worlds of desire. One is mommy and one is wife, yet both strangely make me feel that I am not quite enough for either. When it comes to acknowledging my husband's desire, I am not a cheerleader. Because what makes me satisfied now is just getting kisses on the cheek from my son. Even after I know he has picked his nose just before that kiss. That is somehow more pleasing than any other kisses I got from all the boys I ever kissed.

But my love for Hayden and Tyler is so intertwined: Without this man, I wouldn't have my little one. Hayden is so smart and funny. He's original. He's caring. Hayden is the Tyler I met and fell in love with, and they have the same dimples when they smile.

. . . .

On my second date with Tyler, we went out for brunch near the hospital where he was working as a surgical resident. He'd been on the breast cancer rotation in his general surgery training, and he told me the story of a patient he had just treated. He couldn't get her out of his mind.

"She didn't speak English very well. I speak broken Spanish and I figured out that she had a lump in her breast and it was growing. She had been to two other clinics and they told her that she was too young to have breast cancer. But I was worried about the lump. So I did a biopsy and it *was* breast cancer. When I did the mastectomy, the cancer had spread. It was too late." His voice dropped and his eyes got teary. "The worst part was that she had come in with a little boy. . . ." I started to cry too. "Sorry if this is too depressing. . . ." He reached across the table to grab my hands and squeeze them hard. "There's this amazing woman who works on the breast service. She's a social worker and she'll sit for hours with patients who are going through a diagnosis. She helps them so much, much more than I ever can. It's pretty amazing what she does for these patients. You have to meet her."

I respected how Tyler loved working in the clinic, and how much he wanted to help people by being a doctor. I loved that he had a pager. It was annoying that it would always beep during our dates, but to me it meant that he was a part of a bigger world. He was responsible and devoted. It didn't hurt that Tyler's blue eyes matched his blue surgical scrubs and his shoulder muscles were bulging against the sleeves. It didn't hurt that this humanitarian was a major hunk. There were a lot of things making me fall in love with this guy. He seemed so grown up—I was only twenty-two, hoping to go to graduate school for journalism, and he was actually saving lives. I pictured him performing a mastectomy, and how sad and complicated it would be for this young man of twenty-six to remove a young woman's breast in surgery. I had always thought of surgeons as being so steely, like the scalpels they used, but this guy was crying about a patient he couldn't help. The fact that he wanted me to meet this social worker he admired so much meant he respected women, and he wanted to share with me something powerful about his job, not only the medical part, but the hope.

Years later, the story Tyler had told me about the young patient with advanced breast cancer would save my life. Eerily, I had my mastectomy the day after I turned twenty-eight, the age of the woman he had treated. It was Tyler who got me to start performing breast exams. I didn't know anyone with breast cancer, but he'd name all my friends and then say, "One in eleven of them will get breast cancer. It's an epidemic."

As he spent more time in the hospital than he did with me, because of his training, I could see that the stress of taking care of patients and the lack of sleep could be overwhelming. One day we were at the movies and a patient kept paging Tyler about his pain after surgery. Tyler was moody and distracted; there never seemed to be a moment when he wasn't taking care of someone or something at the hospital.

"Why don't you reassure him?" I suggested. "Tell him you're sorry he's in pain, and that you hope he feels better soon."

"That's exactly how I feel, but you really think saying that will make a difference?"

Tyler took my advice, and the patient stopped calling. Tyler was soon ending every call with a patient, "I'm sorry about your pain and I hope you feel better soon." I knew that he respected and trusted me. He listened and that meant so much. It felt like we were a team, supporting each other.

When he proposed to me in 1991, on a freezing night in New York City, he had somehow hidden the ring, champagne, and champagne glasses under his overcoat. He had chosen the winter solstice, the shortest day of the year. We were in a horse-drawn carriage in Central Park. Snowflakes were falling, and the driver had two glowing plastic roses on his carriage. It felt like we were on a movie set, and after Tyler told me he wanted to spend every moment with me for the rest of our lives, he suggested we smash our champagne glasses.

"This moment can never be undone," he said.

We could see our breath on that freezing night. I can still remember the heat I felt in his kiss, against the icy air. I can still remember the shiny glass shards scattered on the cement.

We went to Italy for our honeymoon, in 1992. We kissed so much it was hard to eat the freshly made pasta that was cooked to a texture that wasn't just al dente—it was *perfetto*, with sauces I had never tried before, like salmon Gorgonzola. The wine in Italy didn't give me a hangover; they say it's because it has fewer sulfites, but I think it was because everything was different in Italy. It was a language of *amore*, and we were fluent. We looked across the table at each other, eating our fresh pasta Gorgonzola, drinking our sulfite-free wine, and I couldn't believe how much Tyler loved me. The candlelight only seemed to accentuate his deep blue eyes, which perfectly matched the warm Mediterranean waters. Those Mediterranean-blue eyes were warm and kind, and he only had Mediterranean eyes for me.

It was as if I spoke opera. Every thought, every question, was a declaration of love and passion, uttered in sweet soprano. I remembered from my music classes that the soprano took the highest part, which usually encompassed the melody. We were in harmony; he was a sexy baritone, but a sweet one. Everything I said was a lovely aria, sung to him. He answered, providing accompaniment, only after I had sung. The aria went something like:

"My dear husband, you are so handsome, what's for dinnerrrrrrrrrrrrr?"

He tilted his head slightly and then sang back.

"Oh, beautiful wife, whatever you want, your wish is my pleasurrrrrrrrrrrrrrrrrrrre!"

Everything around us was art, and the colors and scale amazed us. Especially the statue of David, that masterpiece of Renaissance sculpture: seventeen marble feet of standing male nude. Although the statue represents the biblical David, I thought his body looked like Tyler's. My man, all of five feet eight inches, seemed to dwarf the huge statue, and looking at David made me feel a flush for Tyler. Priceless statue of a biblical warrior hero? Sorry, I choose Tyler. I squeezed his hand while our tour guide explained more about David versus Goliath. I just kept thinking about David versus Tyler. No contest!

I can't remember the way we kissed on our honeymoon. I want to go back to Italy to find out again. The only Italian in my life these days is delivery pizza with a map of Italy on the box. Venezia is so far gone. I want to be sitting next to my husband in a gondola, making out and cuddling him, holding him like we'll never want to stop, even if the boat capsizes. *I want to eat Italian food every night for dinner.*

. . .

*T*he operas we used to sing have become couple's therapy sessions, Tyler and me sitting in separate chairs, across the room from each other, trying to figure out how to find common ground. I can't remember the last time we held hands. We have become like other couples we saw on our honeymoon: Married many years, they could sit through a five-course dinner without uttering a single word except to the waiter, usually requesting more vino. Back then we had so much to talk about, and we were appalled that they had *nothing* to talk about. I think of those older Italian couples now, and I think maybe they were being polite, like, "If you don't have something nice to say, don't say it at all." Why do marriages go from dinners filled with witty conversations and kisses to silent standoffs? Theoretically, we should have so much more to say to each other now after so many years together and so many more things in common, like our kids.

On the last day of our honeymoon we wandered into a traveling exhibit of art by Salvador Dalí. The curator, with a French accent, caught us staring at one particular painting. She must have seen us holding hands, and maybe she thought we were an easy target for a romantic story. We were on our honeymoon, or *luna di miele* in *italiano*. It was August, and Italy was crawling with newlyweds on their *lune di miele*.

"Oooooo la la. You have found my absolute favorite print in the entire exhibition. This is Gala, Dalí's wife. This painting was inspired by the first time Dalí ever saw Gala. He saw her back. It was *magnifique, parfait,* and he thought to himself, *I must have this back.* It is pure luuuuuuv."

I was totally in love with every particle of Tyler, so I understood how someone could fall madly in love with someone else just from loving her back. Every bit of Tyler—even his back, lightly freckled, muscular—was dreamy.

"And then Dalí approached Gala, and the rest is history!"

She continued talking with her French accent about all the unique aspects of the print. How Gala was so pure he could see through her, and this was represented by her hollowed-out reflection in the picture. Eros, the Greek god of love, was in the picture too.

The more she talked, the more I realized that I had to have this print because it represented the marriage of "love and desire," as the curator explained, the exact combination I felt for Tyler.

She continued to taunt us with details of the strange but inspired love they shared. We were mesmerized as she explained how Dalí introduced himself to her.

Legend has it Dalí prepared himself for the encounter in a totally symbolic way. He cut himself while shaving his armpit, so he smeared his body with his own blood, mixed with fish, glue, goat dung, and oil. He accessorized with a pearl necklace and a geranium behind his ear. Gala was smitten.

"Dalí had so many pet names for her. Galushka, Gradiva, Oliva for the oval shape of her face and the color of her skin, Oliueta, Oriueta, Buribeta, Buriueteta, Suliueta, Solibubuleta, Oliburibuleta, Ciueta, Liueta. And my favorite is Lionette, because Dalí said that when she got angry Gala roared like the Metro-Goldwyn-Mayer lion!"

I needed this print. I wanted Tyler to think of me as his muse. I was amazed that Dalí thought that Gala was irresistible, even when she was angry.

That curator with her French accent talking about true love and passion really was a tonic. I wanted to be like Dalí and Gala, maybe minus the goat dung and fish and blood. We parted ways with a passionate kiss as I went to shop and Tyler wanted to see more art.

We had discussed whether we should buy the reproduction, but it was expensive: The gallery representing Dalí's estate had stamped it with his name and used high-quality paper and ink. We had wedding money, but the purchase seemed too decadent, even though it would be a honeymoon keepsake we would treasure.

I went back to the hotel to take a nap, regretting not buying the print. Tyler woke me up with kisses and a large cardboard tube.

It was Gala, rolled up, to take home to New York City.

"Promise me you'll always tell me what you want," Tyler said. "Don't ever settle in our life together. I know you wanted that print." I was so blown away by the romance of the gesture.

. . . .

*W*hen we got Gala to New York, my uncle in the framing business recommended an art framing shop.

"Let me look," said Patrick, a very distinguished type of older gentleman who wore a silk pocket scarf in his blazer as he unrolled the print in his frame shop.

"Ah . . . Gala!"

I was so excited that he knew about Gala. It just added to my joy in having her. She must have been more famous than I realized.

"I worked with her in the theater in New York City."

Tyler and I couldn't believe our good fortune, meeting someone who had actually known the woman in our print.

He started to take out samples of all the gold frames that would match the gold-flourish details Dalí had painstakingly added to decorate Gala. Patrick paused and looked directly into my eyes.

"She was a real *bitch*, you know. She drove him crazy, not in the good way."

. . .

*H*ad I become Gala?

It's hard to figure out the imperceptible changes that add up to where we are now. If I were to create a flipbook, starting with our drunk-on-love wedding pictures and ending with our couples-therapy faces now, would I be able to find the moment where did the change happened? When did we stop being a team, and start taking opposing sides about almost everything? Why is the beginning picture so different from the latest one? If my engagement ring could talk, it might warn me that it wouldn't sparkle as much after almost twenty years, and it would definitely look smaller as my finger and pant size expanded.

Our big twentieth anniversary was only a few weeks away. Tyler had sort of blown off the past few anniversaries. They weren't nearly as romantic as the honeymoon, and I was dreading the inevitable letdown. Tyler had stopped buying me jewelry because he claimed I always returned it. We would make a romantic date night, and inevitably a kid would get sick.

I remember when it was all so perfect. I remember when we celebrated every month we were together. I remember when it was hard, when I was in chemo, and we even tried to make it perfect then. Tyler had taken me out to lunch for a romantic date, but I was so tired I fell asleep on my plate and got quiche in my hair. At least we tried.

I remember when we spent so much time choosing the perfect gifts and cards for each other. I remember when I googled a list of anniversary presents given for each year, as an incentive for Tyler. Technically, I reminded him, we were on china. What would we do with fine china these days? We heated up our meals in the microwave. There were a lot of take-out containers and macaroni and cheese, and none of the fine dining we did when we were dating. China felt so impractical for our current status; platinum was the modern gift for a twentieth anniversary. Tyler reminded me that my wedding band was platinum, and that I didn't wear it anymore, so why buy another platinum ring? I had outgrown my ring. I seemed to have outgrown the romantic symbol of that beautiful platinum ring too. We had become so practical as life plodded on. Life had become predictable, so far away from the Tuscan hills of Italy. There was so much paperwork, school forms to send in, bills that arrived every day.

. . . .

*W*e had scheduled a meeting with our insurance agent for the night before our anniversary. She was reviewing our policies, and Tyler said, "I've been thinking about it. I want to buy Geralyn a long-term-care policy." Our insurance agent looked at Tyler and looked at me. She had helped me to get a life insurance policy after my breast cancer. She knew how much this request meant. Not only did Tyler think that I would live long, but that I might even outlive him. He wanted to make sure someone would take care of me. She pulled out a stack of forms. "This policy is about to be discontinued because it's so good that they're losing money on it. This policy will cover Geralyn until she's a hundred and twenty. That is a very thoughtful gift."

They say diamonds are forever, but I think a long-term-care policy actually might be the closest I'll ever get to forever. I want to live until I am 120 and I think, for the first time ever, that *maybe*—just maybe—I'll die of old age instead of cancer. Tyler had always believed that I was cured and I would live. I sort of resented him for that, because it felt like he was trivializing my pain and fear. But maybe he really did believe I would be okay. Spending money on a long-term-care policy was quite a vote of confidence.

I was almost tempted to ask our policy adviser what would

happen if I died young and didn't need the long-term care. Would Tyler get a refund? I didn't want him to waste the money, but then I realized it was a good bet to place: a bet on living so long that I'd need assistance to keep living. I liked the ring of it. I liked thinking of myself as a Long-Term-Care Policy Holder.

I love my husband. He always promised to take care of me, and I'm touched that he is worried about what will happen to me when I get old. I'd never thought of a long-term-care policy as a romantic gift: It's a different type of love from the honeymoon-opiate type, but it's fine. It is *long-term*, like the health-care coverage. It is more solid and thoughtful than any set of china.

My relationship with my son is evolving too, into a more mature love. The other day, when I told Hayden something, the boy who used to hang on my every word said, "Mom, who asked you your opinion?"

Actually, Hayden is having an affair and cheating on me . . . with Tyler! He has left the Oedipal phase and entered the "identification" phase, and he's totally besotted with his dad. He sleeps tucked under Tyler's arm every night. I am no longer between them; Hayden is now between my husband and me. I nurse my heartbreak, and there is a small upside to his new infatuation with his dad. Seeing my little guy look up to my big guy has sort of shamed me into remembering why I fell in love with Tyler in the first place. Watching Hayden absolutely idolize my husband and want to be him so desperately has made me put on my rose-colored glasses again for Tyler. I made the right choice. He's a good man and a great father. He's taught Hayden how to walk, how to sled, how to ski, and a lot of other things too. Hayden wants to do everything Tyler does, exactly the same way.

He's started leaving the toilet seat up and even started criticizing me at the grocery store. "Mom, why do you think we need more milk? You never finish what we have and then we end up throwing it out."

It was true love all around.

CHAPTER 11
Sweet

*A*fter cancer, celebrating my birthdays is a little bittersweet. Of course there is huge relief I've actually lived another year. But birthdays now make me aware of how much every year is truly a present, one I might not get to open with as much joy the next year. I'm not quite sure how to celebrate them anymore. Sometimes I hide and try to pretend the birthday isn't happening.

But today I decided to shake it up and take my fears head-on. I'm sitting in a tattoo parlor, wearing a flashy "Sweet Sixteen" blinking tiara, a tight black bodysuit (with Spanx underneath), jeans I had to lie down in to zip up, and a push-up bra that sort of makes my post-mastectomy reconstructed rack work really well. The tiara is awesome: It has a battery switch in the back that makes the entire tiara light up hot pink and then makes it blink extra-hot pink intermittently. "Sweet Sixteen" is written in pretty script across the top in gold, accented with really big blingy rhinestones. The tiara is perfectly balanced on my head, held in place with combs that dig into my hair, which I just had blown out after I had it dyed to hide the gray.

I'm *so* not sixteen.

Even though I'm in my midforties, today is my *cancerversary*—sixteen bonus years since the day of my mastectomy. It is strange that my birthday and mastectomy date are only one day apart, but my doctors refused to operate on me on my actual birthday; they didn't want me to associate my birthday with the operation. I wasn't convinced at the time that there would be many more birthdays because my tumor was so aggressive and I was so young, but I was wrong, and so were the doctors who thought my prognosis wasn't good.

Even though I have survived sixteen years, every cancerversary feels like I have just been diagnosed again. The triumph of the cancerversary is always a combo of bitter and sweet: The pain is still so fresh from my trauma, but the joy is there—that I am still *here* . . . wearing a blinking "Sweet Sixteen" tiara *and* Spanx. I am surprisingly grateful for the muffin top I have grown over the years; I am grateful for my a-little-bit-mean-to-her-mom tween daughter; I am grateful for my husband, even though we are in couples counseling; I am grateful for my son, even though he's becoming sort of grumpy like my husband. I *am* grateful for my life.

But I am still scared of losing the beautiful and messy life that has been my second act after the cancer. I have much more to lose now if it comes back: my healthy body, my gorgeous daughter blossoming into a woman, my prince of a husband who puts up with me, my completely original and freethinking son.

I've come to a tattoo parlor because it's a place where people *choose* needles and pain, where people smile after the pain, so different from the hospital, where I am forced to go for my checkups and scans to make sure the cancer isn't back. I am always scared of my cancer coming back—but right now I'm more scared of the woman behind the desk at the tattoo parlor, because she has full tat sleeves up both arms, along with a large sparkling nose ring. I am brave, but not that kind of brave. She's given me the tattoo book to thumb through to pick out what I want. The friends who have come with me are sure about their choices, but I'm not: one is getting a gator, the other, a survivor too, is copying my winged heart on her reconstructed breast and inking a girl boxer on her arm.

I'm going for something much more subtle and personal than an entire arm sleeve or a dragon: I have decided to get "HEALED" spelled out across my butt in elegant curlicue script letters. I considered doing it on just one cheek, but that felt too noncommittal. I want this to be an announcement, a declaration, a billboard of sorts. Tyler gave me his approval, and no one else will see it—but *I'll* know it's there.

A lot of survivors celebrate their treatment-completion dates every year. Some have parties, some go on cruises, and some prefer quiet reflection. Quiet reflection? Not this year! It's my *Sweet Sixteen*!

I've ordered myself a fabulous birthday cake and I am not going to share any of the icing roses. And I brought champagne, because I can drink legally at this Sweet Sixteen. Madonna is blaring too. Happy cancerversary to me!

Under the hot lights, with beautiful tubes of inks and the buzzing of the tattoo needle, I'm feeling bold. I'm giving specific instructions to my tattoo artist, Josh, whose kind green eyes make me feel so centered until I notice the snake crawling up his neck.

"I want the tattoo to spread across my butt, like one of those banners the airplanes pull across the sky at the beach." I'm trying to be clear and really explain how artistic my vision seems. "Like it's unraveling its message. Sort of an energy to it."

Josh is totally getting the vibe. I'm a little self-conscious because airplane signs seem tacky for invoking a moment as somber as declaring my total cure.

Airplane signs usually advertise beer specials at "Ladies' Nights" or "No Credit Check" car ads for new leasing agreements. Maybe I need to elevate my vision. A banner is too obvious, like I don't actually believe I am "HEALED," like I am trying to advertise it or prove it to myself. Maybe a small, tasteful, lower-right-cheek tattoo might be less embarrassing if I end up back in the hospital for cancer treatment and my gown opens up in the back and my butt accidentally peeks out.

I say the word out loud: "Healed."

Josh nods his head.

"I love the way it sounds. So definite and elegant and safe. It's like a stamp we're putting on my body to prove I've crossed over to the other side and escaped the cancer shadow."

Josh is really deep in thought for me. He's been the consultant on my other three tattoos, but this one seems most important, the final statement. I got the first tattoo at the lower end of the diagonal scar that crossed my reconstructed breast: a heart with wings to remind me to live with courage and to remind me of the angels I'd met. I got the tat instead of a nipple, to show myself that nothing would ever be the same again. I couldn't just "replace" my nipple, and the winged heart was a symbol that my new life would look different. I thought very carefully about how down the road some mortician might view that mastectomy scar, and how the tattoo would symbolize hope and maybe make the mortician smile: She would know that I had found a way to decorate my scar and love my wound.

My next tattoo was a wing behind my left shoulder, like an angel looking over me, dedicated to a friend who died of breast cancer and left behind a little boy. She had always wanted a tattoo of angel wings, but her white blood cell counts were too low from her chemotherapy. A group of her friends went and got tats for her as a tribute after she died.

My third tat was two stars on my left wrist, one for each of my kids. Those tattoos were videotaped for a YouTube video I did called "Ouch," to show women that getting a tat hurt more than getting a mammogram.

I can hide those star tattoos under my watch at parent-teacher night. In fact, I can hide all my tattoos so people don't judge me. I'm pretty sure that I used to judge people with tattoos, and now I have three, going for a fourth. My friend was a bit worried about this tattoo thing—was I moving into fetishism? I'm a bit worried too, in the tattoo parlor, about getting inked again. But I'm certain that *this* tattoo will complete me.

I think I am finally ready to move past my past. I think the healing has finally happened. And writing "HEALED" across my butt will be different from writing "CURED." Whenever I read an article about a celebrity who declares herself "one hundred percent cancer-free," I wonder how she knows. Who is her doctor? Is she taking new patients?

Cancer cells are so small and all of us have them at any moment. It's up to the fighter cells to stop them, and somehow my fighter cells had lost their fight before. Do my fighter cells have game now? Am I truly healed? I might never be cured—that felt way too certain and definite. Being "HEALED" was more of an evolution and a state of mind.

I chose the word because I remembered a speech an oncologist gave at a cancer luncheon in New Mexico, about what it meant to be healed. I was so curious about when a person knew she was genuinely healed. Was there a test? Could she prove it to me? "Many of my patients consider themselves healed, even when they're dying" was her answer to my skepticism. I looked at her like I didn't believe her—how can you be healed when you're dying?—but she looked right back at me like she didn't care if I believed her or not, because she had some truth that she didn't need to prove to anyone.

As I am telling Josh the story of why I picked the word, just saying the words "healed" and "dying" together make me a little teary. Something about the word *healed* is making me think of so many unhealed wounds.

I ask Josh if I can take a moment because I'm feeling a little dizzy too. I sit down on the tattoo table and gulp some of my cancerversary champagne straight from the bottle. Instead of relaxing me and chilling me out, thinking about being healed is having the decidedly opposite effect on me.

I chug more champagne, and it's as if wounds start oozing out of my mind: boyfriend wounds, professional rejections, friendship falling-outs. *Healed* is a word that is so provocative, that feels so unfinished for some reason, especially now.

Should I get a question mark after the word? It might be more authentic. But I can't walk around with an unanswered question on my body.

Josh sees my tears and is reassuring. "Let's do this!" he says. I hike my underwear down a bit and get ready to lie over the table.

Josh is patient and totally feeling my dilemma, exactly as engaged as you want your tattoo artist to be. Part therapist, part painter, the tattoo artist has to manage fleeting emotions with permanent ink. I have seen the laser therapy needed to remove unwanted ones. Choosing a tattoo is much more important to me than choosing paint for my walls, a new carpet or sofa. Josh is my personal exterior designer, and we can't choose wrong.

All my tattoos have stories, and I need this story to be as true as the others. He starts to make other tattoo suggestions. Anything goes with Josh except getting a guy's name on my body. Josh has had to fix one of those for a very famous client. I know that Tyler would be horrified if I had *his* name written down there.

Suddenly I can't hear a word Josh is saying to me. He looks like he's speaking in slo-mo, because I am lost in thinking about how to heal my heart after my tragedy. What kind of bandages work? How do I move on? I picture the Band-Aid from my childhood knee scrapes. The sting of the antiseptic spray before the Band-Aid went on, knowing that underneath there was some process going on, something strange and magical, so that when I took off the Band-Aid there would be fresh, clean skin growing over the wound. There would be a time to take it off, and all would be okay.

．　．　．　．　．

*M*y huge faded-red mastectomy scar seems just as fresh and tender now as it was at first. All these years later, I walk funny, holding one side of my body back protectively so no one can brush against me. My scar is a souvenir from that trauma. It is the badge I wear every day. *I will never be healed.* I will pay tribute to my trauma. I will live my life as fully as I can but *I am not healed.*

I still wince when I think about the day the bandages came off and I was nervous to see myself for the first time. The wounds took longer to heal than I had expected; doctors always underestimate the pain factor. Every time I thought the bandage was dry and the wound was healed, it would weep just a bit more to remind me not to get too cocky. The bandages are long gone, but the wound is still fresh in my psyche. I am so vulnerable, yet I want to live like I own my life. How do I tell the story of wanting to live even while I'm scared I might die? How do I make *this* tattoo's story the one that explains how I feel about living? I stick my finger in an icing rose.

I feel like Cinderella, dancing at the ball, but the clock is ticking very loudly, reminding me there's a deadline when my dream might unravel. I want to live. Just let me live. Maybe that is what I should have Josh write? But is it too obvious? That has been my wish on my birthday candles every year, as well as in the machines I inserted my body into to see exactly what was happening. Today I will make the same wish over my sixteen candles. I was lucky because my chemo worked—it's as simple as that.

I had plans for my life before cancer, but cancer uprooted my plans and taught me that all I have is *now*. But right *now* I want *more*. I want to keep living a lusty life: Sixteen years aren't enough. Give me more. Please. Maybe my plan should be to let my life just hatch—no plans. Plans are for people who have time on their side, and certainty.

Emboldened by my second chance, I decide there is only one choice. I hike up my pants farther to protect my butt from the tattoo mistake that almost happened. I'm *so not* healed. I'm way too ambivalent for that type of declarative statement.

"Josh, could you just write 'Sweet' in a heart on me?" It is my Sweet Sixteen. I have a sweet tooth. I like talking in a sweet voice. I know that life can be bitter, but I want to remember to taste the sweet.

I'm feeling so confident.

"Not on my butt." I show him exactly where I want the heart. I want it drawn above my actual heart, to remind me it is still beating, despite my doubts. Josh makes the heart outline first. He looks so serious, and pauses to wipe away a bit of blood. I see the blood on the gauze, and it reminds me to be brave. The heart symbolizes my courage to face uncertainty. I learned when I chose my first heart tattoo that the root of the word courage is *cor*—the Latin word for *heart*. In one of its earliest forms, the word *courage* meant "to speak one's mind by telling all one's heart."

"I'm going to freehand the word too; is that okay with you?" Josh usually sketches out the tattoo design and then traces it onto my skin. He has just drawn the heart on me, no practice. I'm trying to figure out how exactly he'll write this word freehand in such a small heart, about the size of a quarter—one small mistake could ruin it. It hurts a lot when he presses the needle into my flesh, and there is a weird smell, but then there is a rush of euphoria. All the endorphins kicking in to action.

This is how Josh draws it: with flourish, with complete abandon and total precision. He is so in the flow of his work, and it looks like pure joy. That is exactly how I want to live my life, the way Josh draws "Sweet." I decide to make a choice that going forward I will look for the sweet, today on my strange second-chance Sweet Sixteen, and every day.

I want to get out of the shadow of my past and believe in my future. Now that I have tasted the appetizers of life, I want it all. I want to stick around for dessert and an after-dinner drink. I've gotten greedy about life, lusty. I want to *live*. I want to learn to live in the moment and appreciate life without worrying that it might vanish.

I think about the mortician again, but now she is squinting to read the word "Sweet" because it is so small. She might have to put on her reading glasses for this one. I guess it's good that I'm choosing a less obvious and more mature tattoo in my "older" age, and I laugh.

Can I stay in the sweet? Can I make sure to remember that I chose the sweet even knowing that the bitter can turn up at any moment, without warning? Life had become more sweet since my diagnosis because I saw that it was so precious and fragile. I couldn't choose my wound, but I can choose my word: *sweet*. If I forget to taste the sweet, it is there in permanent ink to remind me.

CHAPTER 12
Bitter

*J*ust as my skin starts to peel off to reveal the fresh ink underneath—
that wound is healed—my cousin Hallie is diagnosed with stage 4
breast cancer. She is only thirty-nine years old. Though I kept my
game face as best I could, sitting with Hallie and her mother at these
first medical appointments was a frightening reminder of my own
cancer diagnosis and the absolute terror I felt in those early weeks.

Hallie had done everything right. Because her mom had had
breast cancer, Hallie had her first baseline mammogram in her thirties. After her mammogram, when Hallie was thirty-eight, she received a letter: "We are pleased to inform you that your results are
normal." Her gynecologist's office had called with the same news.

But, the radiologist had noted on a report that "the breasts are
extremely dense which lowers the sensitivity to mammography." That
one sentence was never shared with Hallie. Her "normal" mammogram had missed a cancerous tumor, which had continued to grow.

My cousin was misdiagnosed and missed a crucial window of
early detection.

Here are three things I want you to know about Hallie before I tell you about her cancer:

1. She renamed herself Hallie when she was eleven years old. Her "real" name is Leland. She is daring like that, even taking on a new name. (I hated my own name too, but it never occurred to me to rename myself.)
2. She is one of the smartest people I've ever met. She started collecting words when she was thirteen, when she read *War and Peace* and discovered the words *hussar* and *bivouac*. (Who reads Tolstoy at thirteen? My cousin Hallie.)
3. She is beautiful. She looks like a mermaid with long, wavy blond curls and eyes the color of the sea. Her cancer treatments would take away her hair, but they couldn't take away her fierce intellect and adorable laugh. I wish I could describe how sweet her laugh is.

Hallie's grandmother Rose and my grandmother Ruth were sisters. They were always very close, even living in the same condo complex in Florida when they were older. Hallie was like my taller, blonder little sister. Her green-blue eyes looked like Ruth's and Rose's eyes. I have brown eyes and always joked that I couldn't believe we were all related. But Hallie and I shared a diagnosis, at remarkably young ages. Was that our mark of relationship?

Years after I was diagnosed but before Hallie was, Hallie's mom, Lynda, was diagnosed with breast cancer when she was sixty-two, and Lynda's younger sister Wendie was diagnosed when she was fifty-nine. When I was with Hallie at one of her early meetings with an oncologist, the same oncologist who had treated me, we drew our family tree. (I hate how genetic history is called *pedigree*, as if we were dogs in a show.) I was the first bad leaf on the tree, and then the other cancer leaves had sprouted. I'd always thought of family history as what came *before*. Now I saw that one bad leaf could signal *future* problems for the tree.

At that meeting the oncologist asked, "Has anyone in your family had ovarian cancer?"

Aunt Lynda said, "My mother did, but she was eighty-one years old."

The oncologist shook her head. "A relative with ovarian cancer at *any* age is a risk factor."

And as if this wasn't overwhelming enough, the doctor also wanted to fill in the other side of Hallie's family tree—her dad's side—because there were significant instances of breast cancer on that side too.

The doctor stared straight at Hallie, Aunt Lynda, Aunt Wendie, and me. "This is a very compelling family history. It doesn't matter what your genetic tests say. Especially with the ovarian cancer."

I wanted to reach across the desk and grab the genetic chart she had just drawn. It wasn't like I wanted to blame the messenger, but sometimes there's no one else to blame. I'd rip the chart to shreds and throw the bits at the doctor, like snowflakes landing on her head. I wanted to tell her that my great-aunt Rose was the sweetest woman ever and that she had always served me cookies and called me "darling" and was so glamorous even in her robe and high-heeled kitten slippers. I wanted to tell this doctor that Aunt Lynda had won an Emmy for writing a soap opera that the doctor was probably addicted to, that Hallie could beat her at Scrabble any day, that Aunt Wendie had hung out at Studio 54 back in the day and had worn better outfits than Cher. This doctor knew only our defects; she didn't know us, and that didn't seem fair.

I started worrying more about my genes, feeling so weird that they were preprogrammed and that I had absolutely no control over them. I used to think that drinking green juice might protect me from possible future cancers, but juicing seemed totally out of this league, where fate made the decisions. And of course, I worried about Skye's future, and I pictured her drawing her family pedigree one day: I'd be the bad leaf that her daughters and her daughters' daughters would fret about. I'd cause worry for future generations because of my cancer. I wanted to pass along only good genes, like the laughter gene and the dance gene. Of course Skye would say I definitely didn't have the dance gene, even though I do. After all, she is on a hip-hop team that wins platinum at state championships. "Where do you think you got those moves, Skye?" From your mother. "Where do you think you got your breast cancer risk, Skye?" From your mother.

By the time Hallie was diagnosed, the genetic-testing revolution had arrived, and I wanted to know if I had the breast cancer gene so that if I did I could have my other breast and my ovaries removed as a precaution. This new blood test analyzed DNA to find mutations in certain breast cancer susceptibility genes. In my test there was a strange mutation called P1238L, which was categorized as "potentially harmful." Years later, Myriad Genetics, a diagnostic lab, would write to my doctor to tell her that the "potentially harmful" mutation had been reclassified as "not harmful." But I wasn't off the genetic hook yet: There was a newer, more advanced breast cancer gene sequencing that my doctor thought I should do because it was more sensitive than the old test. I had it done, and it didn't show anything new. But then there came a *newer* test called BART that could show a DNA problem that might not have shown up on the earlier genetics tests. I did BART and there were no red flags.

It seemed like our family didn't have "the gene." Hallie had all the genetic tests done and hers were negative too. But it didn't really matter what the genetic tests said because breast cancer had now shown up in two *young* women in our family.

At a famous New York City hospital where Hallie, Lynda, my mom, and I have come for a second opinion, the doctor explains Hallie's diagnosis in more detail.

At first there was hope that even though the tumor was big, it hadn't traveled anywhere else in her body. That was short-lived. The bone scan showed that it had traveled to her spine. The evidence was so tiny, almost invisible on the films. There was debate over how to proceed with her treatment. Some doctors suggested ignoring the hairline cancer on her spine, and treating her breast cancer as if it had not spread, as if she were curable. Others had said she was "treatable" but not "curable." This is a sort of code-speak for cancer patients and oncologists, which I'd had to learn the hard way when they thought my cancer had metastasized to a lung lobe. "Treatable" is a way of saying they will keep trying treatments for managing the cancer, but there is no hope of a cure—buying more time but never truly getting your life back. Whether she was treatable or curable would determine the course of Hallie's treatment. Hearing these words again reminded me of how unfair cancer is—how so much of it is bad luck.

This doctor has come highly recommended, and we are all leaning forward in our chairs to make sure we hear exactly what she has to say about Hallie's prognosis.

"You are clearly in the stage four bucket."

I can't believe her choice of words. Bucket? She has to be kidding. Does she not know the phrase *kick the bucket*? There's even a movie, *The Bucket List*, about two terminal patients. I hate the term *bucket list*. The visual of a dirty bucket holding a list of to-dos before dying is so depressing.

I am snapped back to reality by Hallie.

"But another doctor I saw thought chemo might work." Hallie is challenging the doctor, and the doctor is getting more agitated.

"Doing chemo would be a Hail Mary now," the doctor says.

"What is a Hail Mary?" my aunt asks. As Jews and non–football players, we don't understand the term.

"It's when you just throw the football into the air and hope for a miracle—when you have nothing else to do," the doctor replies.

There is a stunned silence. I clench my teeth as hard as I can. I've never wanted to physically harm a cancer doctor—they are my heroes—but there is something evil about this woman.

I look over at Hallie. I wish for a moment that she was the one with all the power, delivering the news to the cancer doctor, and that my sweet cousin was cancer-free. I keep scowling at the doctor, as if I were in second grade, and I wonder what Hallie will do with her remaining time. I remember when I thought my cancer was going to kill me, and I thought of all the things I should probably do before I died. But despite having cancer, or maybe because of it, I never did sit down and make that list.

It gets even worse, if possible: Hallie says to the doctor, "I read that I can have a five percent chance of living."

"It is more like one percent," the doctor snaps back, staring directly into my cousin's stunned eyes.

I try not to cry in front of Hallie that day in the hospital when she is put in the stage 4 bucket, and there's a very clear end date—like an expiration date on a milk carton—stamped on her. When we leave the hospital, we walk across the street and order margaritas. We make a toast to life.

I need to believe in life. We are going back for Hawa's final scan, to see if her cancer has returned. Her sister has flown in from Africa, and we are waiting for Hawa's oncologist to walk into the room holding the film he will put on a white bright light to show us Hawa's future.

It is so quiet in the room; we are all holding our breath. We hear the rustle of the film coming out of its paper holder. The film is glowing mysteriously.

"There is no evidence of disease. You are cured."

We jump and scream and cry and hug and almost suffocate this distinguished and kind doctor, in his white coat, the three of us.

As Hawa is walking out of the hospital, she pauses.

"I need to help Hallie. Cancer survivors take care of each other."

"Will you be scared?"

"No. You taught me to be strong, and now I can be strong for Hallie."

Hallie is determined to live as long as she can. In fact, I've never seen her so determined and hopeful. Despite her dire diagnosis, she is planning for the long term, and buys a new apartment. Her life has taken on a certain "do it *right now*" quality. She makes her new apartment her dream place, spending hours picking wall colors and building in special bookcases to display her prized collection of books. She's ready to find the man of her dreams too. She's been engaged, broke it off, kissed some frogs, and she's afraid that her diagnosis will scare off the dream man—but she flirts with the physical-therapy guy during sessions for her swollen arms. Hawa is determined to keep Hallie looking toward her future. She makes Hallie dress up and put her wig on before the cute physical therapist rings the doorbell.

"Hallie, where is your lipstick?" Hawa and Hallie crack up before Hallie answers the door.

She reaches a milestone and turns forty. In a packed bar, with her friends and family, she sings a Madonna song, "Ray of Light," and dedicates it to her grandmother (on her dad's side), who died of breast cancer. She is singing about pain, the pain of losing her grandmother to breast cancer, and also her tentative future. I can still see her singing that song, perfectly in key (Hallie attended LaGuardia High School of Music and Art and Performing Arts—the *Fame* school). It seems like she is singing to us about how much she wants to live. She looks sexy, fierce, and alive. The crowd goes crazy for her.

White hospital hallways are so much different from a rowdy bar. With each appointment she has for treatments, she is getting further away from the Madonna-singing bar girl. Soon Hallie is spending more time in the hospital than out of it. I try to be strong and not cry around her. I've made a rule for myself about not crying in front of her. But I hated it when people didn't cry in front of me when I had cancer; I thought they didn't care. Now I know that they didn't want to make me sadder than I already was.

Going back to the cancer ward to see my cousin, I smell the sterility mixed with heartbreak, and I am so happy that I didn't get the "HEALED" tattoo—because the shadow is back in my life. During one of my hospital visits, Hallie is told that the treatment isn't working *again*. The nurse says, "Henry Ford had to keep trying, to get to Model T, and he had the entire alphabet behind him in failed cars. You have more options." But we all know she is running out of options fast.

I bring Skye to visit her, and we are both scared when we walk in. Hallie is bald from her chemo and can't speak because her throat has been radiated to shrink a tumor. The cancer is spreading faster than any doctor predicted. There is a huge burn mark on her neck that is red and painful looking. Skye is so poised; she gets water for Hallie and brings her tea.

Hallie whispers, "Skye, I can't believe you're with me today. You must have so many places you'd rather be with your friends. I remember when I was thirteen."

We leave a little later, and Skye looks at me and says, "Mom, I think Hallie is going to *make it*."

How can I pop Skye's balloon of belief? In the elevator going down, I turn to my daughter. "I brought you here because I wanted you to see that I can't leave it. Cancer will always be with me, Skye."

She nods and seems to understand perfectly, way beyond her thirteen years.

Every day of my life is a day *outside* the hospital. Yet being back *inside* is now more familiar, as if I've never left that world of pain. I feel like a traitor getting to walk out of the hospital, leaving my cousin so I can return to the other world.

Hallie is trying as hard as she can. I hate it when people say that patients "beat cancer." Trust me, if anyone could "beat" cancer, it would be Hallie. If anyone could outsmart cancer, it would be Hallie. If anyone could out-charm cancer with her wit, it would be Hallie. She would sing another Madonna song that would make cancer weep and retreat.

Hallie was there with me at my chemo, and I want to be there for her. When I was first diagnosed, Hallie made me a mixtape and wrote on it, "You're not a cancer survivor, you are a *thriver*!" So I am praying for a miracle. Like how I got pregnant and how Hawa lived. Hawa's cancer is gone for now; her treatment has worked. But instead of thriving, Hallie keeps getting worse. And my old wound is fresh now with Hallie's pain.

After one sixteen-hour surgery Hallie has to recover in the wound-healing unit, and when I visit her, everything is so quiet and there is white gauze everywhere.

Hawa has been helping Aunt Lynda care for Hallie during the endless hours in the hospital. She has brought fresh puree food she has made because she remembers how hard it is to swallow after throat radiation. She is guarding Hallie's bed, making sure the nurses and doctors bring her pain medication whenever it is time for a new dose. I'm there with my mom and brother, in this alternate universe. It feels like we are on a space station. Darkness and high-tech machines beeping everywhere. I stare out the window at the Williamsburg Bridge, stare into the night where the city looks like a jewelry box. The traffic lights are green emeralds and red rubies; the white streetlights are diamonds. Hallie can't wear the jewels—they are all in the world behind the glass, far away, outside her grasp. When I look at all the lights, I imagine how the world will continue the next day and people will go to restaurants, taste delicious food, ride in taxis, laugh, but she will be stuck in the hospital in pain.

I want to smash the window and connect those two worlds again for her. She's trapped inside and can't get back into the other world. I cry over her bed. She rustles a bit, but she doesn't realize I am crying. Maybe if I don't cry, we can both deny this is really happening.

After watching her sleep for an hour, my mom and brother and I go out to dinner. I hate leaving Hallie in the hospital. I want to stay there with her. Everyone in this restaurant seems so happy, oblivious to all the people in the world suffering from cancer treatments. I order champagne to make a toast for Hallie, but when it arrives I can't even lift the flute. I just stare and watch the bubbles rise up and then pop on the surface. *That's how fast life happens. That's how busy we all are until we realize it can all pop.*

I put my head down on the table and start to wail and heave. I can't pick up my head and face the inevitable: Hallie can't ever get better. My mom and brother try to comfort me, but then they start sobbing too. When it was happening to me, I didn't have to watch from the sidelines and feel so helpless; I was in there facing chemo and fighting it. I wish I could do chemo for Hallie. I want to take some of her pain away, but I can't.

"I'll never finish my documentary now," Hallie tells me one day in the hospital. For almost two years she's been working on a film about her father's acting career: *Jan Leighton: Man of 3,000 Faces.* I know how badly she wanted to finish that documentary. She wanted to write other books, find a guy she loved, help support the peace process in the Middle East. But her time is running out.

"Before I die, I do want to pass this law that would make it mandatory for doctors to tell women with dense breasts that they need more testing than just a mammogram. There's a piece of legislation now in Albany, but they haven't been able to pass it. I'm going to testify, and I'm going to call every official who needs to vote on this."

Hallie had heard about the legislation from a group called Are You Dense, founded by Dr. Nancy M. Cappello, who was diagnosed with advanced breast cancer despite a decade of normal mammograms. She had passed a law in Connecticut, and was spreading the word that similar legislation was stuck in committee in New York. Hallie starts a blog called *Inform Women* to keep everyone posted on the legislation's progress:

Wednesday, May 30, 2012

Greetings. This is a blog about sausage making, as they sometimes call lawmaking. It's actually about a particular sausage: bipartisan New York Bill S6769/A9586 (Breast Density Disclosure and Insurance) which is in the process of being both made and unmade in Albany. It's a bipartisan bill requiring that women with dense breasts be notified by mammographers that their breasts are difficult to read by mammogram, and that they should discuss additional screening options with their doctors. Right now, women with dense breasts are not informed that they are in danger of misdiagnosis. Women like Joann Pushkin, whose cancer grew for five years undetected by mammogram. Some cold, hard facts: According to the American Cancer Society, in the United States, 40,000 to 45,000 women's breast cancers are missed on mammograms every year primarily due to breast density.

- Ten thousand women a year die of cancers that were missed on mammograms (because of breast density) back when the cancers would still have been treatable.
- A similar law that passed in Connecticut has doubled the detection rate for women with dense breasts who received sonogram screening. So we know this bill will save lives of New York women.

The bill may never make it to the assembly floor. There is less than a month left in the legislative session, and it's still stuck in committee, where lobbyists and legislators are quibbling over the language of the bill. Among them are people who would like to kill this bill without leaving fingerprints. They can do it by running out the clock. With all the procedural hurdles this sausage has to go through, it may not make it to the assembly floor. That's why I started this blog. This sausage can only be cured with some sunlight. . . . There are villains in this story too. At the end of the month, we'll know who the biggest villain is. The winner will get the "boob of the month" award from this blog.

Hallie has researched all the members supporting the bill, and those opposed. She is a fierce self-taught lobbyist. She travels to Albany to hold a press conference and e-mails her friends and families the information of all the lawmakers to call and write to about supporting the legislation.

Hallie tells me she knows she will die. I want to reassure her that she has more time, that she shouldn't think about it. She is brave, though, and on a mission once she's focused on what she *has* to do in her remaining time. Hallie's bucket list is to get legislation passed and make sure this never happens again to another woman. When she grants interviews about the legislation, she always says, "This bill will not save my life, but it will save someone else's."

One day after I leave Hallie and the hospital, I decide to do some research because I probably should make a new, definitive bucket list. Her determination has reignited the questions for me: What do I want to do with my one life? What will truly make me happy? What will I regret if my cancer comes back? What will make me smile if I know I checked it off? What am I missing that will make my life feel even more worth living? Shouldn't I have figured out by now exactly how I want to live my precious life? Shouldn't I be telling everyone to live every moment like it was his or her last?

I should be a poster girl for bucket lists because I survived cancer. But I'm worried mine won't be original or exciting enough. I'm worried it will feel trite. On the other hand, I'm so sick of seeing people jump out of planes just to cross "jump out of a plane" off their bucket lists. I mean, if you can die in a skydiving accident, what is the point of putting it on a list of things to do before you die? Doesn't that defeat the point? I've heard people say they want to run a marathon before they die. Not to be dramatic, but I think I would rather die *than* run a marathon. I have asthma, and I am not an athletic girl at all. Or, again, I might die while running it, only to defeat the purpose of the bucket list. The same goes for running with bulls in Spain.

There is one sport I love, and to be perfectly honest, I have only one thing on my bucket list aside from *living*: shopping. When I was going through chemo, I so badly wanted an adult Make-A-Wish that would pay my credit card bills. But shopping feels shallow now. I need important things on my list; this is life and death.

I decide that I would rather keep Hallie's legislation goal and my list in fancy purses, instead of in buckets. It seems so much more dignified and less dire. Instead of gross buckets used for cleaning dirty floors, our "purse lists" would be pretty, sprayed with a favorite perfume. I do some research. There is a website to help me plan and track my very own list, with ten thousand suggestions. The problem: None seems important enough to be part of *my* purse list:

Eat bull testicles.
Be in a music video.
Ride an ostrich.
Meet Oprah.
Hold a huge spider.
Shave a coconut.
Float in the Dead Sea.
Dive with sharks.
Go grape stomping.
Have a wild deer eat out of your hand.
Eat kangaroo meat.

Okay, I need to stop. There are too many strange animals here. Nothing is rising to the level of an "I must do this before I die" feeling, except meet Oprah.

Maybe my list isn't very daring, but the "shave a coconut" suggestion is making me feel more confident about my hopes and dreams. I just want to live now and get to keep everything I got after cancer. My kids were on my purse list before. Is that enough? Here's my list:

Stay alive.
Never go through chemo again.
Live long enough to see a cure for cancer, but until then, keep
      Hallie and Hawa and everyone sick with cancer alive.

Watching Hallie get through her treatments with such courage shames me. I need to take more chances, bigger chances, live as if each breath could be my last. The ante is so high, and for some reason I'm not rising to the challenge. I don't want to ride an ostrich; I don't want to stomp grapes. I can't think of anything grand enough to prove how much I want to live. I'm having a midlife crisis, and it feels wrong. I have lived long enough to start taking life a bit for granted again, and life is losing its luster. I am alive, but not alive *enough*. I want to fall in love with life again, and remember that it is a present to unwrap.

CHAPTER 13
Blood, Sweat, and Tears

*T*here are things in my life I can't control, and things in my life I *think* I can't control, and things in my life I *can* control. And then there's my ass. My body had betrayed me before with cancer, and now with the twenty pounds I've gained in my forties.

Recently my ass went rogue and knocked over a bowl of spaghetti and a cup of coffee. I was squeezing between two metal tables in a teeny tiny restaurant to get to the seat my friends had saved for me. Like a street cleaner, sweeping things indiscriminately in its path, my ass swiped away the contents of the next-door table as I tried shimmy into the seat.

It was a sign. Actually it was a billboard: I could ignore my ass no more. It craved attention and had a mind of its own. *I* thought I could make it to my seat without disaster, but my ass knew better. I was in denial, hugely underestimating the actual girth of my butt, and the restaurant incident was really just recognition of truth. There was a time when I could have made that squeeze and even made it look cute. I could have taken a deep breath and lifted my ass up a few inches to clear the space elegantly. But now my metabolism was shot and I had lost control of my ass.

From T & A I had been reduced to A, so there was a lot riding on my A. Before my mastectomy, I had looked at reconstructed breast photos in the plastic surgeon's office, to see what my breast would look like after the operation. I was especially obsessed with how big the scar would be. There were different ways to reconstruct my breast: taking tissue from my stomach (there wasn't enough tissue; I didn't wear Spanx back then); my back (ouch); or my ass. I was intrigued by the ass option until I saw a picture: The tissue removal looked like a shark bite on the right cheek. *No way*, I thought to myself. *If I'm forced to have a big red scar on my breast, I must preserve my ass. Keep that scalpel away from my ass.*

"A" had become some sort of last vestige of my womanhood. After I saw that picture, I promised my ass it would be a priority. I *needed* my ass to make me feel normal and whole, like no one would ever cut off a piece of me again.

None of my cute jeans fit anymore. I bought a pair of jeans in my old size: I couldn't pull them over my thighs. I gave them to my friend Christina with the tags still on them, and she could tell I was admiring her ass as she squeezed in. They fit perfectly. When I was forced to buy a new pair of jeans that would actually fit, I finally admitted that my ass was growing like a weed. The saleslady was blunt: "You need the Honey Booty Cut," she said. I had this immediate image of Pooh Bear eating so much honey that he got stuck in Rabbit's front door and couldn't be pulled out. Had I been eating too much honey? I thought about what I had been eating, and knew exactly why my ass had grown so much: meatballs.

"Come with me to my trainer," Christina said. "I'll give these back to you; you'll fit into them soon. Kate is amazing."

Christina didn't explicitly tell me she was taking me to the gym because of my ass; she said that she wanted me to start getting healthier.

To be honest, my current exercise regime consisted of lunging to pick up the Legos that Hayden dropped everywhere on the floor. My other toning activity was reaching across the bar for another glass of wine. I did hop onto bar stools. And if I am to be absolutely honest, putting on a Spanx was the last time I had worked up a sweat and overexerted myself: There was something really wrong.

I don't think it was entirely my fault. My nursery school report card said, "WILL NOT PUMP ON SWINGS," in caps, and suggested a meeting with my parents to discuss the reluctance. There was no under-lying psychological issue: I wanted to get pushed because it just felt bet-ter. Pushing off and starting the pump was way too hard, like biking up a hill. I only wanted the ride down. I wanted the "Wheeeeeee!" but not the legwork it took to get there.

My DNA is not exactly athletic. There were hunters and gather-ers, and I am probably a descendant of another group called loafers, who supervised the entire hunting and gathering going on. I imagined my ancestors observing the hunters and gatherers: "Good job, every-body! When's it time to eat?"

And I'd been reluctant to invest in my health after cancer, too scared of being let down. I'm also intimidated by Christina's gym. It's very industrial, brightly lit, with hand-sanitizer dispensers everywhere, reminding me that here everyone works hard and sweats. The ceiling is high and there are mirrors on the no-color walls. The smell of sweat and then a whiff of laundry detergent from the stacks of freshly washed towels hit me. Equipment is lined up around the room, hangs from the ceiling, and lies on the mats in the middle of the room. There's no way I can pretend this is going to be fun and games. Most of what I notice in the gym, though, are the skinny asses, in black Lululemon leggings, taunting me. I don't trust that my body can be healthy and strong after cancer.

I hear a negative voice in my head saying, *You do not belong here.*

The negative voice is always with me, doubting everything I try to push myself to do. But today it is almost screaming at me that I will fail.

I'm not a gym girl, but I want to stay for Hallie. I want to *move* as a tribute to Hallie, in honor of her, and do things that her body won't let her do anymore. I want to work hard for her. Hallie needs blood transfusions now, which means hours of sitting in the hospital hooked up to an IV. I remember those long hours of sitting and waiting, from my own treatments. Being in a gym is the furthest thing from being in a hospital. Survivor's guilt doesn't even begin to explain my emotional state; I have survivor *trauma.* But I still need to be strong for her. I feel inspired to take myself on after watching my cousin be so brave. I want to control my body.

I haven't jumped rope since I was eight, so when Christina's trainer, Kate, hands me a jump rope, memories flood back—of getting tangled in the rope with Jane when my friends Robin and Diane turned. I was a better turner than jumper. Now I am reluctant to jump rope for Kate because maybe I've forgotten how. Plus my ankle hurts because I sprained it in a pair of high heels, and I have to explain to Kate that I've injured my ankle not doing sports but doing fashion. I start to jump and instantly I feel like I might pee in my pants. I can't hold it in. I jump three turns and have to stop. Kate looks at me like she's been expecting lame, but this is really capital *L* Loser Lame, and I blurt, "Sorry, I need to pee."

"Don't worry, that happens to all my women clients who've had babies." Her voice trails me into the bathroom.

Kate is a cross between Mike Tyson and Paris Hilton. All brawny and girly at once. Her arms are humongous, but so are her boobs. Her legs seem lumberjack, but her lips pout. She is always sipping water with Crystal Light to stay hydrated, and eating protein bars to bulk up even more. She also has flowery tats on her super-defined back. She grabs weights with her manicured nails like another woman would grab a purse. Kate scares me.

I want to stay in the bathroom forever, but when I come out and Kate hands me the rope again, it hurts to jump. I can't catch my breath. The voices in my head are asking me how I got so out of shape. The rope is too heavy and I trip over it because I can't make it go fast enough. I want to quit and sit down and chill. I want to go home and crawl into bed and stay as far away from that jump rope as possible. Christina is jumping fast, almost skimming the floor. I can't keep up! But Kate is staring at me with her heavily eyeliner-lined eyes.

"StairMaster," she says.

She holds out her bulging arm for me to grab as I climb on. I'm sure I'll fall off, and Kate looks a little worried too. Do I look down at the stairs rushing toward me, or do I look ahead because I'm getting dizzy? How do I make this machine go slower? How do I turn it off? Stairs keep coming at me, faster and harder. I keep stepping but I'm getting disoriented and even dizzier. Make the stairs stop!

"Kate, help!" Kate hits the clearly marked button right in front of me, and I jolt to a hard standstill. I stumble off the StairMaster and Kate points out the step-off step I've missed. Christina jumps on and starts running up the stairs.

Kate hands me a kettlebell. "Push it over your head and bring it down."

I start imitating her motion but then the weight of the kettlebell almost topples me over to the right, so I swing it to the left to compensate—and then Kate intervenes.

"Whoa, whoa there. Coming down with the weights is as important as pushing up. Control is key. Control."

You've lost control over your life, not just your ass, that voice says.

I want to take that weight—the kettlebell that looks sort of like a Kelly bag purse with a top handle—and throw it, maybe shatter the mirror, smash the floor. Maybe they'll ban me. Maybe I'll never have to come back here and lift this metal thing that is making me hurt and shake. I just can't push through this pain. I am more exhausted from this than from any all-nighter I ever pulled in college. I am so thirsty, I could gulp an entire huge bottle of Gatorade like those jocks on the commercials.

Kate is not letting me off the hook. She thinks I can do things that I know I can't do, and that I'm holding out on her. She keeps saying things like "Come on, I know you can do this." But I know I can't. She has more confidence in me than I do.

Kate will soon figure out that you can't do it.

Next I have to pull these rubber band straps—called TRX, which hang from the ceiling—back and forth as hard as I can and pretend that I'm rowing. She makes me do fifteen reps. I want to tell her that my arm is still weak from my mastectomy, all these years later.

You just want an excuse.

I ask if I can get water, which I figure will give me a little break, but Kate says not until number fifteen. I take the longest water break ever. I am guzzling water as if I were a camel in the desert. "Water break over!" Kate screams from the other side of the gym. "And fill your cup so you don't have to keep going back." Christina smirks at me like she might have tried the water trick too, when she first came to the gym.

The way Christina got me here was by saying, "Just try it for three sessions. If you never want to come back, you don't have to." Forget three sessions, Christina. I don't think I can last even this one.

Kate takes me, Hannibal Lecter–style, down to the basement, which has a contraption with weights on it that she wants me to push along a strip of fake grass that stretches the length of the gym wall. It's called a sled. I try to push it forward and I can't. I have pushed a baby stroller, a full shopping cart in the grocery store, and an overflowing cart at T. J. Maxx, but I have never pushed anything that looked like this. I want to be pushed, not push. "Keep going. Push!" Kate is in my face, moving along next to me. I am walking, not running, and I am hunched over trying to find something inside me to help me push. I finally get to the end, with relief—and Kate tells me to turn it around, switch poles, and push it all the way back to the end again. "Faster!"

You are not really strong; you know that.

After that, Kate has me lie facedown on the floor with my forearms flat and parallel, and push up to a plank position, sort of like a push-up. She makes me hold the position, and my whole body starts to shake. I'm supporting my weight on my forearms. I collapse after about a three-second hold.

"I want you to get to fifteen seconds on holding this plank." Kate starts counting again. Her face seems distorted as she is counting down because I am seeing dots and I feel sort of blurry. All I can hear is "Three, two, and . . ."

"Just say 'one' already! Just say it!"

I plop onto my stomach with my head down. I want to stay on the floor forever. Christina has already sprung up, and she throws me a towel.

"See you *both* on Wednesday," says Kate.

Christina pats my back. "Try it two more times, and you never have to come again."

I come back on Wednesday, mostly because I don't want to disappoint Christina, and Kate tells me, "On the treadmill walking for a five-minute warm-up."

Suddenly I feel compelled to tell Kate everything I have eaten the night before: "Meatballs, pasta, and three glasses of white wine." Kate seems truly grossed-out, like this is an epiphany of sorts for her.

"We have to get you eating right. Protein every two hours. No more drinking alcohol on weeknights, only weekends." She is going on and on about how I should be eating grilled chicken or fish with salad and I don't hear anything about meatballs, even in moderation.

After pounding on the treadmill for five minutes, I am already tired.

Kate, for effect, adds to my pain: "And all of that work is not even a *lick* of those meatballs you love." I feel so hopeless. I don't want to give up my wine and meatballs, but just walking around in high heels isn't keeping off the calories that the wine and meatballs are putting on. I want to announce to everyone in the gym how hard this is for me. That I don't belong here. That it's all a mistake. That I am more comfortable at my favorite Italian restaurant called Parma, just three blocks away from the gym.

And then I hear her. "UghaaahaaaaAHHHHHHHHHH!"

She sounds like she is either getting beaten up or having an orgasm. I can't help but look, and in the middle of the gym there is a woman with the kettlebell above her head. Every time she lifts it over her head she makes that sound. Half grunt, half scream, fully distracting—I can't stop staring. She continues to make so much noise doing her workout, it's embarrassing. She growls, she moans. . . . Such a strange combination of pleasure and pain.

I'm so jealous that she is fine with making these animal sounds in the middle of a packed gym. I have a horrible habit of putting a smile on my pain, and the Groaner is showing me that maybe there's another way. I am in awe of her. After her workout she crouches in a fetal position, which is exactly what I want to do after my workout, but I've been trying to keep my game on. I decide I want to show my pain more; maybe it will help me manage my agony. The next time I meet Kate and Christina I try it out.

"UGHAHH?" I try to groan with the same intensity of the Groaner.

"What was that?" Kate looks concerned.

"I'm trying to manage my pain . . . with groaning."

"I think you're either a groaner or you're not." Kate seems to take her role as my adviser very seriously, and she doesn't want me humiliating myself any more than I already have. I love her for that.

Working out still hurts and I still can't keep up with Christina, much less with Kate, but I do keep showing up.

Just skip your workout. Just stay the way you are. It's easier.

Slowly I am able to function a bit better. I make sure to pee *before* I jump rope. I can do the five minutes on the StairMaster without tripping. And I start to tone down the grunts. I am expressing the pain, feeling it, being it.

I am so sore after four sessions of training that it hurts to sit on the toilet when I pee. My body is in shock and so am I that I keep going back for more sadism. I am so tempted to sleep in and eat a doughnut instead of going to the torture-chamber gym. Every session brings a new form of pain.

Kate teaches me to do a push-up correctly, and I have newfound respect for Michelle Obama. I am not allowed to dip my head and I am not allowed to keep my ass in the air. "Bring your butt down with you. Put it down! Take your butt with you."

It becomes our ritual that I start every session on the treadmill, panting, telling Kate what I have eaten the night before. It is sort of like being in the confession booth. Kate went to Sacred Heart and her mom is Catholic, so she is down with it.

"I had Chinese food last night." I still pant even at just five seconds.

"Chinese is a great option!" Kate seems excited, like I might have made a good choice. "I go across the street and get steamed chicken and broccoli."

"I had lo mein, and an egg roll, and—"

Kate puts up her hand to stop me. Her eyes wander to my ass, and I think she can see the egg roll settling in. But working out is making me really hungry. I want to quit so badly, because I don't see any progress.

When does change actually happen? *You are still the same.*

I want to feel that exercise high that so many celebrities brag about feeling when they work out. I just feel exhausted, and I look the same. Maybe I should do Pilates instead because I'd get to lie down on my back while I was exercising. This boot-camp type of exercise is really too hard for me.

Christina got me to the gym, but it's my decision whether or not I'll stay, and I decide I'm going to break up with Kate. I come in with my breakup speech, but Kate is smart. She says that I need to have a private session with her.

"I want you to run on the treadmill today instead of walking."

You were just going to dump her; she can't make you run.

And then I start to jog.

"Faster, and *don't* hold on to the side!" Kate is yelling at me.

I let go of the side rails and I'm sure I'll fall over sideways, but I am running, sort of. The belt keeps going, and I don't fall off.

"Get your speed up." Kate is pushing her red-manicured fingernail on the button, in the up direction. She's watching my numbers and I start to push myself really hard, and the number of miles per hour are creeping up. She arches one Botoxed brow as best she can and says, "I think we are having a breakthrough."

"Kate, do you feel like my therapist?"

"Nope," she says confidently, "I just *make* you do things."

"Good job." Kate hands me a towel. "You're coming a long way."

Ha, five minutes?

I remind myself that when I first came in I was out of breath after five seconds of *walking*. I feel such a rush of accomplishment. For the first time in my life, I feel like telling my negative voice to shut up!

I usually listen to my negative voice; it usually wins. Yet I know that I am slowly getting stronger. Kate tells me that she's adjusted the length of my TRX bands because she thinks I can handle more resistance. I don't think I can.

I can.

I start to cry, and I turn away from Kate. "Sorry, I just can't believe that I feel so strong. My body feels like it can finally do things."

I think about what it means to be strong. I can't remember the last time I felt strong. I picture myself lying in the hospital bed after my mastectomy, when everything hurt. I couldn't even smile because it hurt the muscles in my face. I remember how still I had to be when the chemo was being pushed through my veins. The needles hurt so much. I was tired and weak, and I wanted to sleep all the time. I remember how I couldn't stand up after my C-sections. It was hard to walk just one lap around the hospital floor. And it still hurts where they cut me, especially when Kate makes me lift a huge ball up into the air while doing a sit-up. I still hold my body defensively, on the right, as if wearing a bandage over my chest.

Could my body be strong for me now? Is this strong for real?

Don't let your guard down. Your body betrayed you once.

Just as I am beginning to feel strong, I hear that Nora Ephron has died of cancer. I didn't even know she was sick. I got to see her genius up close when my story was part of a play she wrote with her sister Delia. I saw how funny and fierce, how alive she was—she became a role model to me. My story was about my cancer, and it had a happy ending. But now *Nora* is gone. And if someone as brilliant, successful, clever, driven, and powerful as Nora could die of cancer, then I am screwed.

I am feeling anything but fierce when I walk into the gym the morning of Nora's memorial. I have a session scheduled with Kate, which I usually dread, but today I decide to push myself harder than I ever have, to honor Nora.

I feel as if I'm transforming, like the Incredible Hulk, turning green with rage. Every step of the StairMaster, I think about how Nora can't climb stairs. Every reach of the TRX equipment, I think about what Nora would say watching me look so ridiculous pulling on these giant rubber bands. But I pull hard for her.

I turn to Kate, who is watching me. "Push me harder, Kate. I need to feel this workout hurt more so the other hurt goes away. I want to do more."

Even if I hate it, I know I am lucky to be moving, to be working out so hard. I'm not in an OR bleeding from a scalpel, not in a hospital gown waiting anxiously for the result of a scan. I am alive. I am in a smelly, sweaty gym, making my heart pound with exertion and adrenaline, reminding myself that I am alive and this is the pain I've chosen. This is my pain now. This lunge, this awful StairMaster, this jump rope that makes me pee, will *cure* me in their own ways, even if my cancer comes back. My fear of the cancer returning is driving me to become stronger.

Through the pain I remind myself of Hallie, who now needs a cane to walk, and of why I am here even though I still feel like quitting every time I'm in the gym. Am I so lame that a gym would intimidate me after I've stared down cancer? So I connect to that mastectomy-and-chemo courage and I use it to push me forward. I have encouraged my kids to take risks, my friends and family. . . . Why can't I? Why can't I believe in myself?

You are lazy; you had no choice with your cancer. You won't choose to keep coming to the gym. This is a fad. You will lose momentum and go back to being you.

My friend Tomomi, a young cancer survivor, knows I'm trying to get fit, and she invites me to do a spinning class at SoulCycle with her. It's the morning of the Race for the Cure, and I was supposed to walk. I have done the race so many times, but today I can't face the signs on people's backs, the pictures of the women they have lost to cancer. I so dread the day I will see Hallie's name on a sign.

Studio B at SoulCycle is dark, hot, and sweaty. Cool music mixes are pounding so loudly that some of the riders wear earplugs. There's a disco ball in the middle of the ceiling, strobing, and a mural of the sky on the walls. When I get on the exercise bike, I need someone to help me adjust the seat and the handlebars and to clip my shoes to the pedals. I flash on "WILL NOT PUMP ON SWINGS." I want to be helped. I want someone to actually pedal the bike for me.

Everyone in the room is pedaling furiously, like their bikes might explode off the ground and fly away. And then they're standing up out of their bike seats and still pedaling. I can barely keep up with my ass planted on the seat. Then they're increasing the resistance on their bikes to make it *harder* to pedal! I pretend to turn the resistance up. I am panting and I'm absolutely sure that everyone is staring at me.

You don't belong here, and everyone else does.

I think that everyone is staring at me—but no one is. Is this the truth about my whole life? That I'm trying to stay in step so I don't get noticed—while everyone else is too busy worrying about themselves and too busy pedaling even to look at me?

The instructor tells us to grab the weights behind the bikes. We have to pump the weights while we are pedaling, but I can't do two things at once. I am not following along with the group, in unison. I am out of sync. I go right when they go left. I spy the glowing red

EXIT sign and I want to run out of this class, the way I wanted to run out of the OR on the morning of my mastectomy. That red EXIT sign is telling me I can leave and go back to my old life.

What if you just stop pedaling?

I can't leave the class because I have no idea how to get my shoes unclipped from the pedals. I'm stuck, pedaling, pushing forward. The class ends and I notice that the name of the class is "Soul Survivor." I am a SoulCycle Survivor, and today I like that better than being a breast cancer survivor.

Tomomi brings me back to SoulCycle: "Try it again. The first time is so hard!" I have to ask someone to help me set my bike again. Today the instructor is Stacey, and she is so cool; I feel awkward around her. Stacey looks like Venus in a badass Adidas tracksuit with a cool headband tied across her forehead to soak up sweat. Her eyes are kind, but her energy and voice are loud. She is chill and ferocious and I am under her spell and totally hypnotized by what she is saying. All the negative thoughts I'm having (what if I fall off the bike? what if I have explosive diarrhea? I can't keep up with the class! I am too weak!) are being replaced by Stacey's positive affirmations:

> "You own all your power."
> "You are winning the battle with yourself."
> "Ride sexy!"

Stacey then says, "Have a conversation with yourself *right now*." And I say to myself, *I love you.*

I'm stunned, and the negative voice tries to talk back and tell me everything that is wrong with me, but I can't hear it because Stacey has put on a super-loud mix of techno and pounding disco music, and is shouting, "Dance on your bike!"

I am finally able to lift my ass off the seat and stand up out of the saddle, though I have to quickly sit down again. But at least I've stood. I pretend to turn up the resistance, and instead of looking at my watch to see how much longer I have to pedal, I smile. I'm having fun on the bike and not thinking about how much it hurts or how tired I am. My legs think they can't keep pedaling, but they do. I am dripping sweat, and totally in the sweaty moment. I start to cry and the salt water blends with the sweat on my face and the tears are mixing with the sweat and I taste the hope that my life is changing right now on this bike in this moment. I am so glad that I forgot to put on deodorant. I smell like a locker room, not like perfume, and I am excited about earning this sweat and not covering it up.

Stacey is howling encouragement at the class. "Exercise will change your life. I don't drink caffeine and I don't drink alcohol. I exercise! Close your eyes and see the word 'nothing' in white Helvetica font in front of you."

I close my eyes and the word is there, glowing in front of me. "Everything you thought of when you saw that word, that's what you need to work on right now," Stacey says.

When I saw the word *nothing*, I thought about being strong and how much it worried me that I might slack off and not go back to the gym. What if Kate or Stacey gives up on me? What if I give up on me? I have changed, but now I begin to doubt that it will stick—maybe the change will just be fleeting.

How do I get my change to not change? How do I get it to last? Stacey starts dancing to the disco techno music, and people on the bikes are screaming her name. She is doing a dance that's a cross between Madonna's "Vogue" video and a Native American rain dance. It is so fierce and so alive.

"This room will change your life!" she shouts. "I have seen the change that has happened in this room. It is amazing. This room will *make you better*! It's *magic*!"

I think about some of the rooms that I was sure would change my life:

- the classroom, where I thought that *A*'s would prove who I was
- the room of my wedding ceremony, where I thought that being in love would complete me
- the operating room where my cancer was cut out, and I was sure that no future problem would bother me if I could just *live*
- the labor and delivery rooms where I held each of my children for the first time and thought that being a mother would give me purpose
- my office, where I was convinced that making money would show me what I was worth

In each of these rooms I looked for the EXIT sign, ready to move on to the next thing. Now I am ready to stay. This SoulCycle room has become about more than sculpting my ass. Finally I've showed up—not for my parents, my husband, my children, my friends, my doctors, or my employers, but for myself.

Virginia Woolf said that every woman needs a room of her own. At that time she meant a room with a door to close, a space for quiet reflection. Virginia could never have imagined that my room would be filled with sweat and bikes and pulsing music. There is no agenda on the bike except for health and joy, and I am riding for *me*. I've waited my whole life for this moment: I am in the room for me. Women had to tell me that I deserve my own room. Thank you,

Christina and Kate. Thank you, Tomomi and Stacey. Thank you, Virginia.

I can finally ride a bike standing out of the seat for forty-five minutes. I still can't do the resistance and I still pretend to turn the knob, but I have learned how to adjust the bike. I still sometimes need help getting my feet to stick to the pedals; that's a work in progress. I sweat, and I always cry during the ride because I am on the bike and not sick in the hospital. No one can see my tears because I am sweating so much. I smell so bad. It must be all the wine and Chinese food seeping out of my pores; that's what Kate told me. I don't want to cover up this smell. I think it must also be sadness and fear seeping out. I can't cover it up anymore—I *want* it to come out.

Since Tomomi shared Stacey with me, I have to share Kate with Tomomi. Even though she can whip through a hundred-minute spinning class, she can't lift the kettlebell that looks like a purse or do a lunge.

Kate has us lunging side by side. "Watch Geralyn's form, Tomomi. Stop, watch how Geralyn is lunging."

Moi?

I have *form?*

I think of my first spastic lunge when I almost fell over sideways and Kate had to spot me, holding my hands as if I were a baby learning to walk. Watching Tomomi's struggle reminds me of mine; she is huffing and exhausted and looks so defeated.

"I know you can do it," I say to her, and I mean it. Her battle with the kettlebell makes me see how hard it is to change. Before now I had convinced myself that change came only mentally, because I could never control myself physically. I *want* to work on my ass now, to change something on the outside just because I can. Working on my ass is working on my mind, my soul even. But even so, my ass isn't getting exactly the results I wanted. One session on the StairMaster equals only about one meatball: fifty-nine calories. Kate says she's seeing results, and even Tyler thinks my butt looks more toned. There's a scale on a landing between the floors in the gym, an old-school scale with a lever that dances toward the right until it balances. I spy it every time we go down to push the sled on the fake grass in the basement. One day, before I leave the gym, I step on. The lever keeps jumping like a Mexican jumping bean, right past my old weight.

Am I the only woman on earth *gaining* weight from intense workouts?

"Don't worry, muscle weighs a lot more than fat." Kate has seen my disbelief. "It's about how your clothes fit; trust me, you're losing inches."

I decide that my ass needs a room of its own too. I go up two pant sizes, and now there is much more room to breathe. I don't feel so confined, and maybe I am cheating, but my clothes fit much better, like Kate said they would. I know that it might seem as if I were changing in the wrong direction, weighing more, going up a pant size, and refusing to give up meatballs (though I have cut down on my wine), but Eastern philosophy tells us that change is always happening, even if not as obviously as Westerners would like to see. I know that I am changing.

Just as I am thinking about skipping the gym, I read a new study that says exercising can make people live 3.1 years longer. Working out with Kate and pumping on the bike with Stacey is adding years to my life. I still obsess over dying of cancer, but I like the idea of working out and adding years to *my* side, and—for once—of *me* having some sort of control over my destiny. Me, not the cancer. There is no guarantee, but *trying* for once feels okay.

I am in this SoulCycle room for me. I am inside the room I feel so alive in. I am not running *from*, not running *toward*. I am perfectly in place, enjoying the ride.

And the bike is the only thing that is saving me. The Soul studio is my place to be strong for Hallie, and I even convince myself that if I push really hard in the class, maybe I can transfer some of that energy to her. I know this is crazy, but it's like a fight for life on that bike. The pounding, the sweating. Every time the lights are lowered, I cry for her. I stop wearing mascara to class because if I wear it I end up with dark smudges and tear trails under my eyes, and then when the lights go up again it is too obvious. I push myself harder on that bike than I ever have, as if my pedaling could stop Hallie's cancer from growing.

Rihanna's song "Love Without Tragedy," starts to play, and Stacey tells us, "This song is very emotional. It's okay to cry because the lyrics are about dying in the moment."

The idea of dying in the moment hits me. I had planned my death a thousand ways: The cancer would go to my brain, to my lungs, to my liver. There would be tubes coming out of me, machines keeping me alive. My hair would be gone; my soul would be crushed; my body would be invaded, weakened, and not mine. But here I am on the bike, eighteen years later, pedaling as fast as I can. I imagine smashing through the lines I've drawn for myself my entire life.

My mind and body have met. I'm not scared anymore. I want to die in the moment, and that means I want to live as hard as I can. In this room, on this bike, there is no yesterday, no tomorrow, just the sound of pedaling. The bright red EXIT sign is still facing me. When I first came to this SoulCycle room, the EXIT sign taunted me to leave. But I stayed in the room. I traveled a distance that I had never imagined for myself. I finally believe in myself, and now I want to stay.

Stacey says to the class, "Today you are training like an athlete!"

I'm an *athlete*?

I've never been an athlete or really wanted to be an athlete. But it feels so cool, so new, and so hopeful. I'm training! I have no idea what the hell I'm training for, but watch out: *I am training*. It feels so alive. It makes me want to be a verb. Actually, it makes me want to be a present participle. I remember that from my seventh-grade grammar class: *The present participle refers to things that are still happening. To make the present participle, the ending* –ing *is added*.

I want to keep pedal*ing*. I don't know where it will take me, but right now I am laugh*ing* on the bike. I want to keep writ*ing*, search*ing*, lov*ing*, grow*ing*, chang*ing*.

*Ing*ing.

I got to live, but it finally feels like my life has become about liv*ing*.

Power was taken away from me when I was sick, but Stacey told the class when we were holding the weights over our heads on the bikes, "The power is yours!"

Don't get too cocky with all that power.

Just watch me. I grabbed my power back. And I told the voice again, "Shut the hell up!"

"Connect to the beat. Stay connected. Staying connected to the beat will make you live longer," Stacey says.

I look up, and in the front row I see a young girl pumping on the bike. She looks like my cousin Hallie. She is singing loudly; she has the most amazing voice. She's standing up on the bike, and the edema brace on her arm is gone. She is riding with me, pumping hard and singing. This is the first time in a long time I've remembered what she looked like before she was sick.

"You deserve to be happy. You deserve to feel joy. This is your one life," Stacey says, pushing us as hard as we can pedal.

"Sprint!"

I am pedaling so hard it feels like my bike might fly off the screws keeping it mounted. The tears and sweat are stinging my eyes. I see

Hallie's face. *"Don't worry, Hallie. I'm going to be strong for both of us now."*

Stacey ends the class. "Thank you for showing up."

Even though I divide my days between the gym and hospital, straddling the world of robust health and sickness, on the bike I have fallen in love with life again.

Chapter 14
Honey, You're Never Ready

My cousin has started to suffer so much from her cancer that no medication can get her out of her pain. Every movement hurts. She is in bed, groaning from pain. I go to the Soul studio and make myself groan too, but they're grunts of strength and hope for Hallie.

Hallie tells me from her bed, "Do you know what I miss most? Just getting dressed. Standing in an elevator."

It is so hard to watch my gorgeous long-legged cousin—who passionately loved vogueing to Madonna—using a cane. Seeing her in a wheelchair breaks me on a whole new level.

I hurt so much during and after my workouts that I realize I am trying to make myself feel pain because she does. I can *choose* to have pain in solidarity with her; somehow we're in this struggle together. Getting on the bike and going to the gym becomes a ritual, a way of praying for my cousin. It is my safe space—the furthest thing from a hospital. There are real demands being made on me by Stacey and especially Kate. I have no excuses not to sweat and push myself. I have never sweated so much—it is as if my entire body is crying.

Then one morning I wake up with a crushing pain in my left thigh. It feels like an elevator door is closing on my leg. It starts spasming. And if that isn't unpleasant enough, the left side of my lower back hurts like hell. I am slightly self-conscious, because there is such a huge difference between a backache and terminal cancer that it seems ridiculous even to mention it. I'm embarrassed to seek help for my back, but when Tyler sees me limping and examines me, he insists that I need an MRI.

Tyler takes me to the MRI lab, and my friend Tomomi shows up too. I don't think they need to be there, and I'm embarrassed to be having any medical procedure when Hallie is in the hospital. I put on my lipstick and get ready to go into the MRI machine.

I freeze. It looks like a casket. I can't face going inside it, being enveloped by that machine with no way out. I take a deep breath and force myself to lie down on the scanning table. It slides into the enclosed tunnel, and once it fully covers me, it continues to slide me even deeper into the tube. I start banging for them to stop it.

"Help! Get me out of here!" I'm gasping for air. I have *never* had a claustrophobic attack in an MRI machine before.

"I have to get out of here; I have to have something to calm me down! I need a Klonopin. Do you have a Klonopin?" I've started carrying them in my purse, as a "just in case," but I know my little plastic container is empty. I guess I've had too many of those "just in case" moments, despite my attempts to have a worry-free day.

Someone is pounding on the door of the MRI room. It's Tomomi, and she comes inside the room to talk to me and help me calm down.

"Only ten more minutes!" she yells over the sound of the machine. "You can do it, Ger! Only eight more minutes!" Then, "Only three more!"

I hear her voice and am so thankful she is there. This is how breast cancer survivors cheer each other on and deal with these machines.

The next day I go to the spine doctor to find out the results of the MRI. Sitting in a hospital gown on the examining table, Tyler by my side, I listen while the doctor explains that I have L3 and L4 lateral herniations. That means worse herniation than regular herniation. Tyler winces when he hears the official diagnosis, which is exactly the diagnosis he predicted when *he* first examined me.

The first thing I say to the doctor: "I'm an athlete."

Tyler laughs. "She's not an athlete."

"Stacey told me I'm an athlete, and I'm in training." I believe Stacey. I have never thought of myself as an athlete before, but I do now. I want this doctor to know how serious I am about the bike and the gym. I need to get back to my training.

"Okay, athlete, let's get you back in fighting form."

And what the doctor says on my way out hurts almost as much as the shot he gives me. "No gym, no bike for at least a month. You need physical therapy. Do *not* lift anything or get on that bike," he warns me sternly. He must see the disappointment on my face. What am I going to do without the bike and the gym?

After months, the actual day for getting back on the bike arrives. I'm sweaty with panic and afraid I'll get hurt again. How will my other discs *not* herniate? One wrong move and I could be back in the MRI machine, with more painful shots and more physical therapy awaiting me. I bite my lip to taste my lipstick as I climb back on the bike and clip my shoes into the pedals.

The woman next to me must have seen my ambivalence.

"First time?"

"No. Well, it's my first time back on the bike after my back injury. I'm not sure I'm ready—"

"*Honey*," she interrupts me. "You're *never* ready."

Should I get off the bike? I panic again.

She adds, "Don't worry so much. You're a spring chicken; I'm seventy-one. I've had three back surgeries. I have rods in my back. I'm okay. You gotta get back on the bike! Just get back on."

Then she starts pedaling furiously, as if to prove to me it's my turn now.

I have zero excuses. The music starts pounding; I begin to pedal. Hallie is dying. I do not trust my body. But I *will not* let my fear of getting hurt again get in the way of my life.

I pedal slowly at first. With every move I make I'm acutely aware of the damage I might do. I can't ride like this. There is no joy. I hate being aware of every twinge in my back and of how vulnerable my spine suddenly is. I like living in ignorance better. It is such a burden to understand that the things we take for granted can go wrong.

About halfway through the class, I face the facts: It won't be fun if I'm going to ride scared. I want to hold back and protect myself, but there is something stronger that's urging me to lift my butt out of the saddle. It is like life. If I hadn't had Skye—for fear that the cancer might come back—I never would have become a mom, and learned to be nicer to my own mom. If I hadn't had Hayden because I was scared of my lung nodule—well, I can't even imagine how much I would have missed. I'd been scared to take a break from working in corporate America because it was the only identity I had known, but when my job disappeared I got to spend more time with my kids.

I've had my second act, a life that was cancer-free, but can I have a third? Can my next chapter take me out of the shadow of cancer that still seems to cast its darkness? Can I finally truly pedal forward, knowing I might get hurt, but feel the joy, the sweat, and the heat, and let myself melt into that singular moment, like Mother Teresa advises, without looking back or forward? It was the joy I remembered, before the back injury.

Stacey is screaming at us, "Find the beat! It's *so* important to stay in the beat!" For the first time I feel the beat. I'm in it! I came to work on my ass, but I stayed to work on my heart. The heart is a muscle too.

Hallie is whispering in my ear as I sweat on the bike. She is saying, "Live!" I can only pedal forward.

CHAPTER 15
Good-bye for Now

*O*ur days with Hallie have transitioned from versions of horrible to sad. There is a difference. The horror mobilized us to fight: Fight with the doctors because she wasn't getting enough pain meds. Fight with the oncologists to continue her chemo even though it wasn't working. Fight with the nursing staff because breakfast was taking too long to be delivered or it arrived cold. Sad is when the fight is gone and the inevitable sets in.

Soon it is Passover, Hallie's favorite holiday, the one that she loved to host for our family. So we ask for special permission to have a Seder for our family in the hospital, with her. It's hard to ignore the unhappy contrast between this Seder and the last Passover Seder we had before she was diagnosed with cancer—when she prepared everything expertly, led us in singing as she carried her delicious food from the kitchen, then carried our empty plates back again. She sped from cooking to singing to serving, and smiled the entire time.

Now the scene is the family lounge at Mount Sinai Hospital. Aunt Lynda, Hallie's mom, has run around town in a mad dash to buy all the perfect dishes for this impromptu hospital Seder. Watching my aunt care for her daughter has been the worst part. Aunt Lynda is caring for Hallie like she is her baby again: feeding her, tending to her wounds like boo-boos that she wants to make better. I have watched her cry, "This isn't the natural order of things. This is a cruel joke! This should be me!" Aunt Lynda has rallied to make Hallie's last Seder special: She even remembered the scallions, which were Hallie's favorite touch. In Israel she had learned a special Persian tradition that Jews swat each other with the long scallion stalks at Seders during the singing of the "Dayenu" song.

My cousin is seated in a hospital chair, dressed in her hospital gown but wearing lipstick. It's hard for her to talk because the cancer has gotten to her lungs and she's so short of breath. We are all gathered around her, our chairs pulled close to hers. Hallie has not abdicated her role of leader. She has always been the teacher in the family, the "wise one," even though she wasn't the oldest.

Hallie begins the Seder: "Suffering is so important for what it teaches us."

Her hair has started to fall out again from the chemo that isn't working. Her arm is swollen and excruciatingly painful. The cancer has ravaged her bones now, and when Tyler looks at her X-rays he can't believe the multitude of microfractures he sees.

But she is still beautiful.

The real meaning of Hallie's speech isn't lost on us. She tells us about suffering, and how suffering is part of our heritage and the holiday, how the Jews had been enslaved for so many years in Egypt. Passover, she reminds us, is about the Jewish people finally finding freedom, and we don't miss the parallel: Now Hallie is a prisoner of her cancer and there is only one way she'll find freedom.

If any one of us has doubts that Hallie knows this is her last Passover with the family, she dispels them: "Next year, take time. Don't just rush and throw the Seder together. Really take the time to do it. Be thoughtful about it."

Hallie's time is leaving her, and she wants us to grab on to ours. Hallie is giving me a master class on life and living; she is the most important professor I've ever had. I look around at my family and can't imagine us next year without my cousin.

. . . .

It is hard to identify that line where Hallie's treatment ends and her dying begins. She is having chemo until two days before she dies. Hallie is in love with hope. She loves it when her art therapist comes to visit her. It is as if she leaps into a cloud and is able to leave the hospital behind and do collage for an hour straight. She loves discussing the peace process in the Middle East because she had lived in Israel and is very opinionated about it. She loves discussing her book, *Rare Words,* and I open it up and quiz her on the meanings. She remembers every one. She plays Facebook Scrabble with the family and beats everyone. And she is still wickedly funny. We had been sneaking wine into Hallie's room for cocktails for visitors. One night, an important-looking hospital administrator comes into the room.

"There is a report of alcohol being stored and served in this room. I'm going to have to do an inspection."

Hallie perks up, "Forget the alcohol, there are controlled substances in this room!" She's been taking methadone because every other pain med has stopped working.

I decide to sleep over to keep Hallie company. It is so different from our sleepovers when we were roommates for a summer after college, when we would stay up late laughing, eating, and watching TV. It is totally quiet; the room is dark, except for the red lights on the machines. Tonight it's snowing, a light and beautiful snow, and the lights of the city are glowing like candles. It seems like we are trapped in the sealed little bubble of a snow globe, unable to interact with the outside world, hiding from ordinary life. We have no idea how much time is actually left—is it days, weeks, months? Do we even want to know?

It's ironic that outside her hospital room window at Mount Sinai, Hallie has a perfect view of Central Park. A park she spent her childhood playing in, a park she will never walk through again: She's more comfortable in a wheelchair or her hospital bed in these last days. My gorgeous cousin, with whom I danced just months ago onstage at my daughter's bat mitzvah, doesn't complain or say it is unfair. But that is what I'm thinking as the nurse comes in to take her "vitals," although she is clearly dying.

"I'm a late bloomer, like my mom and dad were. There's so much more I want to do." Hallie is fading in and out of sleep.

Every once in a while a machine beeps, but aside from that there is a comforting silence between us, where she could say anything and we are safe from the crashing reality that starts at daylight when the doctors visit with more dire news and painful procedures.

How will I say good-bye to Hallie? I feel so helpless, and any optimism or delusions we had about her getting better are long gone. The only thing I can do is just tell her how much I love her.

I know I will have to say a final good-bye soon. During one of her awful treatments, I run out of her room and start heaving into a trash can—I am crying so hard that I start vomiting, and vomit pours from my nose too. A nurse in the hallway comes over to check on me.

"How do you do this?" I ask her. "How do you stay here?"

She looks at me and says, as if it were obvious, "It's my job to help make them feel better any way I can."

I don't know how to comfort Hallie in this long last hospital stay, but I am going to learn from the oncology nurse and make my cousin feel better any way I can. I buy her a book called *What I Love About*

You by Me, which is sort of like a Mad Libs, and I have to fill in the answers specifically about her. It is pretty cool how much she loves being told how much I love her. Our love feels very present tense, but is also something that can never be taken away from us. Talking about our love takes us out of the horror of the moment. As Hallie gets weaker, I read her the same book louder, again and again. We both know it by heart, but she still laughs at each page as if it is her first time reading it.

> #1. I love your *EYES*
> #37. I never get tired of your *LAUGH!*
> #47. I am kind of obsessed with your *BRAIN*
> #43 was my favorite: If you were a dessert you'd be *a cheese plate*

The nurse taking her blood pressure stops and asks, with a bit of a New Yawk accent, "Who would *ever* eat cheese for dessert?" My cousin smirks. She has been to Paris. I want to kidnap Hallie from the hospital so we can go to Paris and eat cheese for dessert.

. . . .

I'm awful at saying good-bye. In a tiny ziplock bag I still have all my hair that fell out after chemo. I'm a borderline hoarder and I can't give anything away. I still have all my baby teeth, my college papers, high school papers, my kindergarten report card, all the love letters and birthday cards I ever received. I don't know what I will do with all these things I have saved, but I can't throw them away. I have to do better with my kids. I have to teach them how to say good-bye to things, but I can't throw away any of Hayden's finger paintings—they are so good, and they represent something so deep to me. I'd be giving away a piece of him if I gave away his four-year-old artwork. The hats that I wore during my chemo are sitting in my closet; I can't give them away because it will seem like I am disrespecting that time we shared together. My story was part of an off-Broadway show called *Love, Loss, and What I Wore*. My bra was in the story—a lacy push-up bra my friend bought for me before my mastectomy. I can't throw that away. I still have the negligee from my honeymoon even though I have changed so much it doesn't fit over my reconstructed breast or my ass. I can't part with anything; it makes me too sad. "Let's burn all the notes you got when you were sick with cancer. It will be very therapeutic. We can have a ceremony and transform the energy," suggests my friend who loves organizing. Creative idea, but nope.

I'm too attached to things, so how can I even think about losing people?

I remember my mom's best friend (and my godmother), Aunt Honey, whom we lost to pancreatic cancer. Told she had only months to live, Aunt Honey refused to do chemo and decided to turn her bedroom into a salon. It was a long good-bye, filled with hugs and memories about her life. She wasn't afraid of dying, she told me. My godmother was giving me the greatest lesson in life: She was showing me how to say good-bye. At my last visit with her she was propped up against the wall so she could greet me—standing—when I went to see her. I remember when Hayden and Skye learned to walk, and how hard it was for them to stand. Honey had practiced.

She knew that she wouldn't live to watch her youngest daughter, Brielle, get married that summer, so they moved the wedding up to the winter. What was going through her mind as she walked Brielle down the aisle, giving her daughter away to her husband-to-be? How could Honey give her away knowing that soon she wouldn't be there? How did she find the courage to give this gift to her daughter? She looked tired at the wedding, and she was starting to shrink from the cancer and become so frail and thin. Somehow she found a last bit of energy and grabbed her daughter and they danced one last dance.

What was she thinking when she danced for the last time? Her face was so pained and tired, yet determined to be there for her daughter. The way she held Brielle was a good-bye that said, "I will never leave you."

The last day I see Hallie, she is getting chemo.

"I love you so much, Hallie."

"Isn't it sad that with all the love I have, it can't cure me?"

Hallie is the deep thinker in the family. Why *can't* all our love cure her?

I have brought her a veggie burger; she takes a bite and pauses. "This would be so much better with mustard." She is right. She is Hallie, tasting the most in the little bit of life that remains to her.

Dying is hard work; like being born, it takes labor. For several days we watch over Hallie in the hospital, until we see the last pulsing vein in her neck, and then there is no more breath. Although we have been waiting, the finality of it is stunning.

Tyler is there to officially confirm that her heart has stopped beating.

My aunt Lynda crawls into the bed with her daughter and hugs her baby for the last time before the funeral home comes to take her away. She caresses her, kisses her face, strokes her hair. She doesn't want to let her baby go.

Her body is still there but *she* is gone, and it is impossible to understand how she had just been with us. At the hospital we all ride down in the elevator with her and leave her with her friend Julia, near the loading dock where the hearse has pulled up. Julia wants to ride in the back of the hearse with Hallie to the funeral home.

"It is an honor to ride with Hallie." She doesn't want Hallie to be alone. None of us does.

Julia tells me later that they strapped Hallie to a gurney, and that the woman from the funeral home protected her when the hearse rounded sharp corners, like holding on to a child in the back of a car in a car seat. Julia delivered her to the official watcher in the funeral home. In Judaism it's a tradition for someone to sit with the body, to guard the soul until burial. It feels good knowing that Hallie's friend took that final ride with her, to care for her until the end.

CHAPTER 16
Stardust

*I*t is the most gorgeous spring day; the cemetery is bursting with life. It seems so cruel to see the crocuses peeking out of the dirt, about to bloom, when our flower is being buried. There is a little sign on the plot: HALLIE LELAND LEIGHTON. We are shoveling the dirt onto her grave, another tradition and honor in Judaism. I don't want to leave Hallie here. In my graveside eulogy I talk about Hallie's college graduation, how I traveled to Santa Fe to be with her that day at Saint John's. It was a day when her whole life felt laid out in front of her. Who could have predicted this end? I'm so glad our grandmothers aren't alive to see one granddaughter burying another.

"Hallie, I remember the swing band that played the night of your graduation and how we danced. This is another commencement. A new beginning for our relationship together. We have so much more living to do, you and I together. I promise your life will inspire mine."

We toss flowers onto the top of the mound of dirt. Her friends and I decide in the cemetery to create a "Dare to Be Rare" club to challenge ourselves to do things in honor of Hallie. We can live parts of our lives as a tribute to her.

The memorial service is standing room only—all of her family and over a hundred of her friends from every part of her life crowded into the Society for Ethical Culture. Because of Hallie's role in the passing of New York's Breast Density Inform bill, chapter 265—a new law that says women have to be informed about their breast density when they get mammograms—Governor Cuomo sends a representative from his office to present Aunt Lynda with a symbolic pen that he signed the bill into law with on July 23, 2012. The legislative aide Hallie worked tirelessly with to get the legislation passed reads Hallie's own words, which she had written in her blog the day the legislation was signed by Governor Cuomo.

> I am over the moon, even though it's [a] little bittersweet. This bill will not help us, the late-stage advocates, in any way. It will not improve our odds of survival. It will not reverse our late-stage diagnosis. It will not bring back Teresa, or lessen her widower's pain. But we're still over the moon. We accomplished something big. The bill will improve early detection and save lives. And I can't say there's nothing in it for me personally. The respective senate/assembly sponsors (Flanagan and Jaffee) who championed this bill, legislators who voted for it, and Governor Cuomo could not reverse my diagnosis but in signing in effect said: Yes, you matter.

The service is led by Carrie, a friend Hallie had met at chemo. Carrie, Hallie, and Aunt Lynda called themselves the Cancer Brigade and Spa. I'm sure Carrie was thinking about her own fragile life, but there isn't a hint of it at the memorial. She is elegant, and not maudlin. She is giving Hallie a final gift.

There is an open mic, and Aunt Lynda invites people from every chapter of Hallie's life to speak. One friend says, "Hallie was my camp friend. The thing about camp friends is you don't get to see them a lot and you miss them all the time. I miss you, Hallie." When Aunt Lynda speaks, she says, "I'm not sure if I'm still a mom. I do have stepchildren, but Hallie was my only child." After a long pause she continues, "Yes, I'm still a mom." Everyone claps for Lynda. Hallie's doctor says she's never seen such a devoted mother. Yes, Aunt Lynda, you are still Hallie's mom.

Hallie's cousin's wife sings the *Charlotte's Web* song, "Mother Earth and Father Time," while holding her chubby cheeked, giggling eight-month-old daughter Hallie had loved.

I'd like to think of my life as a movie now, so I can shuffle through the scenes and hit PAUSE and PLAY when I want to, and have control over Father Time so no one is missing or gone. I hit play on my movie to watch my scenes with Hallie again and again: Sleeping in a park when we're visiting Boston in college, because we've lost the key to my brother's apartment. Visiting our grandmothers together in Florida, eating early-bird dinners every day at four o'clock, turning heads in our bikinis. Being messy roommates one summer.

The night after my cousin dies, my daughter and son are watching a documentary about the cosmos. Certain principles are being reviewed:

1. Matter can neither be created nor destroyed, although it may change forms. This must mean that Hallie is still "here."
2. A certain amount of our bodies is made up of the same matter as stars. Specifically 93 percent. Scientists believe that the saying "dust to dust" is more accurately phrased "stardust to stardust."

I google Halley's Comet that night because I want to register the name "Hallie's Comet" for a new production company I'm going to dedicate to her. Halley's Comet is special because it always returns to Earth, every seventy-six years, and I believe my cousin will always be with me. Unbelievably, Halley's Comet comes up in Google News that day. During early May, the Earth passes through a debris trail left by comet Halley. This results in a meteor shower called the Eta Aquarids.

Was it a sign from my cousin of her safe passage? I know that Hallie is going to heaven, but maybe she is letting me know she is already off in the cosmos, that there is order in the universe. I search on the NASA web page and it says that most people describe Halley's Comet as a meteor shower, but it is really a *celestial firework*.

Hallie would appreciate that distinction. She was always attracted to precision in vocabulary. I picture what a celestial firework would look like. Like my cousin. Hallie didn't just go to heaven; she put on a show along the way.

I decide that my first project for Hallie's Comet is "ABC News Goes Pink," to educate women about breast cancer screening guidelines and to encourage them to get screened. I still feel so hopeless that Hallie was misdiagnosed. I couldn't save *her* life, but maybe I can save *another* life as a tribute to Hallie and her purse-list goal.

All the ABC anchors wear pink on October 1 to launch the campaign. Jenny McCarthy even wears a pink bra on *The View*, and we do a live mammogram on-air to demonstrate to women that it doesn't hurt as much as they think. I had made a video to show women that Brazilian waxes, wearing Spanx, dancing in high heels, eyebrow threading, and tattoos hurt more. I want women to spend as much time, money, and energy on their breast health as on their beauty treatments. I get a new tattoo on-air, for Hallie: a speeding comet on my left wrist around my tattoo of the two stars I have already gotten for my kids.

The ABC correspondent who gets the on-air mammogram is forty, and it is her first mammogram, because she had let the prescription for her mammogram stay at the bottom of her purse. She tells the audience that she's been too busy working and taking care of her kids to follow the prescription and make her appointment. Her mammogram, shown on national TV on *Good Morning America*, will make headlines around the world a short time later: She is diagnosed with breast cancer, and the mammogram has possibly saved her life. She never would have gotten it if not for our project. It is completely amazing that she is saved by the mammogram, especially because she has agreed to the screening in the hope of saving one life. Who would have guessed it would be hers? It is also amazing that she has *another* cancerous tumor, like Hallie's, which isn't even detected on her mammogram. Her doctors discover it when they do the pathology after her mastectomy. Other women around the world get mammograms because of the ABC correspondent's diagnosis. Correspondents in Australia do a live on-air mammogram as a tribute.

Having that one woman diagnosed is, I believe, a true sign from Hallie to keep spreading the word about breast cancer awareness and early detection.

. . . .

Shortly after Hallie's death, Skye finds a lump in her breast. I feel it. People always compare tumors to fruit: This is a grape. Tyler says it's probably a muscle. But when he feels it, in full-on-doctor, no-need-to-be-concerned mode, he too is concerned. A muscle could be felt on the other side also, but this isn't symmetrical.

"She has to go to a breast surgeon immediately," he says.

I do the math. We don't have the breast cancer gene, but breast cancer is in the family, and the next generation can have it ten years earlier—I was twenty-seven; Skye is now fourteen. There are three years till she's seventeen, but they seem insignificant. Three years? Is breast cancer her fate now too?

We go to the same doctor who told me I had to have a mastectomy, and now I am in her office with a daughter with breasts. When we are filling out a family history of breast cancer, I hate that Hallie is just someone on paper, someone who has died. On the line where they ask her name and the age she died, I want to write, "Loved to sing Madonna."

In the doctor's office I blink hard to make sure I'm not hallucinating being twenty-seven again, just diagnosed. The doctor examines Skye and does the same kind of sonogram she did to diagnose my cancer.

"The lump is only breast tissue; you're fine, Skye," the doctor reassures us. I must still look shell-shocked, because the doctor puts her hand on my arm and says, "Skye is fine, Geralyn."

When I was diagnosed, my dad told me that he needed to speak with my doctor and ask her a very important question. What he said next stunned me: "Why did this happen to Geralyn?" My father has a doctorate, and his rational mind knew there was no answer to why I got cancer. It was sad that his question was so innocent, like there might actually be an explanation for a tragedy.

"Why did Hallie die?" I want to ask my doctor. But I know I can't ask that question, and the doctor leaves us alone in the exam room. Skye and I breathe and hug. I apologize to her while she is still in her examination gown. "I'm so sorry you have to be here. I was worried when I had you that you might be angry that I had breast cancer, and that you'd worry you'd get it."

"No, I'm not angry at you." My daughter looks confused. She takes off the gown and wipes the sonogram jelly from her breast. She doesn't hide her herself like she usually does in front of me. "Mom, why would you ever think that?"

On the way home in a taxi, we are winding through Central Park.

It is autumn, and the leaves are almost all off the trees. I think about when I lost my leaves, but Skye stops my scary thoughts. "I love autumn when the leaves come off the trees. It makes the park look bigger." She's right. Before I had only seen the naked branches, but now I can see so much more of the sky, vast and unobstructed without the leaves. I think about Hallie playing in the park, and just then Skye squeezes my hand.

"I love you more than any other person in the world."

I am stunned, but I completely believe her.

Skye's breath makes a little cloud in the cab's chill. When she tells me she loves me, it's as if she's blowing stardust on me. Maybe I will be annoying tomorrow, but not today.

We visit Hallie's grave on her forty-third birthday, seven months after we have been there for her burial. The formerly green cemetery is now completely white, covered in snow. We clear away the snow that has covered her headstone: LOVELY, LOVING, LOVED. Aunt Lynda lingers at the grave even though it is freezing out and everyone else is heading back to the car. "I just want to hug her."

This is what I want to know: When does the grieving end and the living begin again? Grief is a gravity field pulling me into the other side with my cousin. One day my cell accidentally dials Hallie's number. There is so much I want to say. I couldn't fit it into a message, but I could tell her some last things: "Your life mattered. I miss you. I promise to never forget you."

Hallie's last book was *Rare Words II and Ways to Master Their Meanings*. Aunt Lynda gave it to me as a memento. On the back jacket there are definitions of two rare words:

Opsimath

Noun. A person who becomes a student later in life.

"An opsimath takes the path of learning late. It's worth the wait."

I am an opsimath: It is never too late.

Funambulist
Noun. A tightrope walker.
"The fun and fabulous funambulist crosses the tightrope (we hope)."

My mastectomy scar has been like a tightrope, a symbol of my divided life.

Cancer and life.

I've been walking on a tightrope with cancer on one side and life on the other, trying always to keep my balance. I try to stay in the middle, but I feel myself swaying toward the world of cancer and fear, of sadness and loss. I've been leaned over toward that side even more now that Hallie is there. But she is sending me a message, ordering me to make a decision right now and stick with it: "Take the leap. Go over and stay on the other side."

Chapter 17
Petal

*T*oday is definitely a Red Lipstick Day.

I'm still wearing lipstick, because the hope I had on the morning of my mastectomy all those years ago has lasted. It's amazing what it means to me now to wear lipstick to my life. Each time I put it on I appreciate that I'm not sick in the hospital, tethered to an IV line. But there are so many more dreams I need to make happen, so many places I want to go—I can't keep track! Every day I dare myself to live up to my lipstick.

Of course, now I wear lipstick for Hallie too, and that feels so important. Whenever I feel fear, I taste that courage on my lips, and I remember how strong Hallie was. She was wearing red lipstick when she was admitted to the hospital for the last time, even though she had a breathing mask over her mouth. I can still see her lipstick-lined lips beneath the mask.

I have to keep living hard for both of us. After what I went through and watched her go through, nothing should scare me in the same way. But things still do scare me, and that is how I know I'm invested in my life.

Wearing lipstick is different for me now: I want to wear lipstick to my life. I think I've finally become one of those ladies I used to watch as she put on lipstick, the ones whose faces said, "Notice me. I deserve this." I believe I deserve this red lipstick too. Life is so "normal" now but not *totally* normal. I'll always have worry, but I will finally try to let go, go with the unexpected, and occasionally take a Klonopin as needed.

I've become a lipstick pusher. When I give speeches now, I ask each lady in the audience to put on her lipstick and make a wish. The wish has to be really big, a Texas-size red-lipstick wish so she can finally see that really big version of herself. It's exciting to watch women overcoming their fear of red lipstick the first time they put it on and reveal another side of themselves. Their eyes sparkle too, with a look of thrill because they've never seen themselves in this way before.

I also make all the women in the audience promise to see only beauty and courage the next time they look in the mirror. These are the first things I want them to see, not their flaws. I tell them about how I saw my own beauty for the first time when my scar was right in front of me, in the topless photo taken after my mastectomy. To see your journey and courage and beauty *first* is a choice.

I've become a red-lipstick counselor. It's ridiculous how so much hope can exist in one small tube. I love to encourage my lipstick-challenged friends to try red, especially at a crossroads in their lives. Maybe it's not cancer my friends are facing, but each friend has her own mountain. Everyone has a wound and everyone has a scar.

I bought my friend Katie a bright red lipstick the morning her ex-husband was getting remarried. I was certain that she would be okay and that there was another fairy tale waiting for her, but I needed to convince her. She was sad, but she didn't know why. Overall, she was happy to be divorced, but she felt the loss, and the uncertainty of the new life that awaited her. I made her put on the red, because it was the first Red Lipstick Day of the rest of her life. She thought she couldn't pull it off, but of course she did. I snapped a picture with my phone of Katie wearing her new red lipstick. She couldn't believe how incredible she looked. And her new boyfriend loved it too.

I can't wait for Skye to grow up enough to switch from gloss to red lipstick. I picture her wearing red lipstick in the future, and her daughter wearing red lipstick, and I will be a grandma in red lipstick. Maybe it will become genetic. A daring red-lipstick-wearing gene, an evolutionary development passed down to new generations.

And then there's Hayden. He placed eighth in the state chess championships. When his shiny trophy arrived, it meant so much more to me than a chess win. I held the trophy and marveled at how improbable it was that I was alive and I had a son—a chess-winning son. Hayden had found his way. A few months later he came home from nationals with a trophy bigger than he was, for third place in the country. Not only was he a chess star, but he was also voted "listening model" at his school for his perfect behavior. His teachers are always remarking on his academic prowess as well as his kindness: "He's the glue that holds the class together" was what they said at his last conference. I'd like to send his report card to some of those awful nursery school interviewers. Not because I'm vengeful—I'm a cautious optimist.

It's nice that I have Hayden now, because Skye is trying so hard to grow up that I don't really see her much. She's always with friends. One night, after she had come home from a hangout and I was asking too many questions, she looked at me and said, "Mom, you have to let me grow up. I need to grow up." Tyler and I can't believe our little girl will be off to college in a few years.

When I was going through my breast cancer treatments, women would always tell me how brave I was. I was courageous, but now I need to learn a different kind of courage—life courage. Slowly I'm becoming a life survivor too. And it feels good. Something totally unexpected has happened between my two scars, my mastectomy one and my C-section one: I've developed some serious abs from my Soul-Cycle workouts.

"Life is what happens to you when you're busy making other plans," John Lennon said to his son. I want to love my life right now. I want to not only stop and smell the roses; I want to take them apart and see the beauty in every petal. Each moment I am living feels especially lipstick-worthy. I have so much more to do—a whole new purse list, and it's *really good*.

I can only pedal forward.

ACKNOWLEDGMENTS

Thank you to my agent, the extraordinary Joelle Delbourgo, for being such a talented matchmaker: I am in love with my extraordinary team at Gotham and know that I am very lucky. Joelle, thank you for your absolute dedication to this project and for being as passionate about it as I am.

To the Gotham team: Thank you for creating this book with me. I deeply appreciate all your time and care and vision. I am so impressed! I am honored to have my book published by you.

Lauren Marino, I knew I wanted to work with you at our first meeting when you took pages of notes and said the smartest things that made me realize what a book whiz you are. Thank you for believing in this project and for helping me realize its full potential.

I'm also so grateful for Emily Wunderlich's pages of fantastic notes (truly) and how much detail and thought was put into our notes sessions. I know your thoughts vastly improved the book.

Lindsay Gordon, you have amazed me already, and we haven't really begun to work together. Thank you to my team: Lisa Johnson,

Farin Schlussel, William Scarlett, Melanie C. Koch, Spring Hoteling, Andrea Santoro, and Matthew Patin.

I became a writer because my former boss, the "goddess" Meredith White, sent pages to the famed Delia Ephron, who supported Meredith's enthusiasm. Delia, thank you for your "blurb" and your incredible support. Thank you for referring me to crackerjack editor Lorraine Bodger.

Lorrie and I worked together on *Why I Wore Lipstick*, and Lorrie has been my architect on both books, entrenched in the process from proposal to end. She knows my voice, sees the problems, but always has the solution. Always. Thanks to Katie Fricas for working so efficiently on deadline with us.

I have also had the privilege of being a writer in Lorrie's writing group, and this has been essential to my process. Thank you to the other writers in the group—Barbara Ginsberg, Ali Perlman, Lynda Miles, Melissa Miles, Jennifer Christman, Robin Rivera, and Ngan Shulman—and thank you to Ashish Verma and Steve Filep for being such gracious hosts for our sessions at the Lowell Hotel. Being around such brilliant writers has inspired me, pushed me, and given me so much courage to tell my story, and I know I couldn't have written this book without workshopping many of the pieces with you first.

Courtney Sheinmel is an amazing friend (we get our breast MRIs together—that is how close we have become) who has become my writing friend/confidante/guru. Courtney says, "I know I am right about this," when she is advising about the book, and she always is. She read every version of the manuscript and had magic solutions. I called Courtney "Book Botox," and I think she is even better than Botox.

My family has been 100 percent supportive of this project, and I am humbled by that support and encouragement. They say that writing a book is like having a baby, so it is fitting that I am writing my thanks on Mother's Day 2014. It is also a miracle that I have become a godmommy this year to Luu Ly.

Another miracle: I'm at the Chess Nationals in Dallas and Hayden has just placed third in the country in K-3 under 800. I know, I'm starting to sound like a chess mom. The trophy is almost as big as now-eight-year-old Hayden, and staring at that trophy is making me a little teary. Some victories are really worth savoring in the moment, and for all the leaps of faith it took to get to them.

This baby, this book, is one of the dreams I want to properly appreciate and acknowledge all the people it took to make it come true.

I never believed I could write one book, and this book, like Hayden, feels like a strange bonus miracle. Here's the secret about a miracle: It needs a team to make it hatch. Although I love to write, I find myself struggling now to find the words to tell you how much I appreciate my family's belief in me.

Thank you, Tyler, for making me a mom and letting me write about you and supporting my writing. You are such a sport, and you have even been a character in a Lifetime movie because of my writing. We will discuss this further in couples counseling. The actor in the movie was really hot, but I still want my real-life husband.

Thank you, Hayden and Skye, for letting me write about you too. It must be hard to have a mom who is a writer. I know one day you will take this book to therapy, but I hope your therapist sees the love and admiration I have for both of you.

My mom and dad, Barbara and Harvey Weiner, read many versions of the manuscript, and my sister-in-law Lori Smith was my first official reader. Lori, your belief in the project gave me the courage to keep writing. Then my other sister-in-law read it. Thank you, Sara Moyn. If two such cool women liked it, I was excited. I guess you couldn't tell me you didn't like it, but I love and respect you both so much. Thank you, Paul and Howard Weiner, for marrying women I really consider my friends too. I am also so happy they kept their maiden names. Thank you to my other sister, Wendy Lucas. And thank you to Uncle Steve for a morale boost and Uncle Marty for your constant belief in me.

I'd also like to thank Hawa Kane, my Senegalese sister, for being a life mentor to me on many levels and for her story of courage. And thank you to Jen DiBella for how you loved and cared for the kids too.

I'd like to thank all my Zeta sisters, especially Nicole and Sherry, for the incredible work you do to support breast cancer awareness, and for including me in that mission.

I'd like to thank fierce and brave survivor Tomomi Arikawa for her encouragement to "write my next chapter" and how much her friendship as a survivor means to me. Thank you for bringing Pink to ABC, which will continue to save lives, and thank you to the ABC News Pink team, especially Santina Leuci, John Green, Adriana Pratt, Danielle Carver, Betsy Berg, and Paul Julian.

There are so many survivors who inspire me through their activism: Thank you to Dr. Marisa Weiss, creator of breastcancer.org; Vixen Marisa Marchetto; Stupid Cancer visionary Matthew Zachary; Courage Night founder Dawn Waltman; cartwheeling phenom Betsey Johnson; Tickled Pink founder Iris Danker; and Dubin Breast Center's Dr. Eva Dubin, for how much you help to inspire other survivors. Thank you to Evelyn Launder for being a visionary.

I'd like to thank my readers and all the amazing women I have met since *Lipstick* was published and became an original Lifetime television movie thanks to Meredith Wagner, who created and led the all-star, award-winning Stop Breast Cancer for Life campaign. Thank you again to Betsy Berg, my speaking agent, who developed the Lipstick tour and always believed my message was larger than what I thought it was. Thank you for the upcoming Life tour. Game on!

I am an author only because I have found my readers, and I

treasure you spending time with me. Readers like Dara Holzman, who reach out and decide to help women, you have made this dream a reality in the biggest way. Connecting with you has been the biggest reward.

And thank you to Stacey Griffith for teaching me that I can only pedal forward in life.

Thank you to Aunt Lynda for helping me share your beautiful daughter's story with the world.

I'd also like to acknowledge the people who will always inspire me, even though they aren't here. My life is better because of you: Thank you, Aunt Honey, Ariel, Joan, Linda, Leland Hallie, Laura, Meredith, Shelly, Nora, Evelyn, Wendy, and Stacey. I miss you.

I will never forget you. *Ever.*